# APOTHĒKE

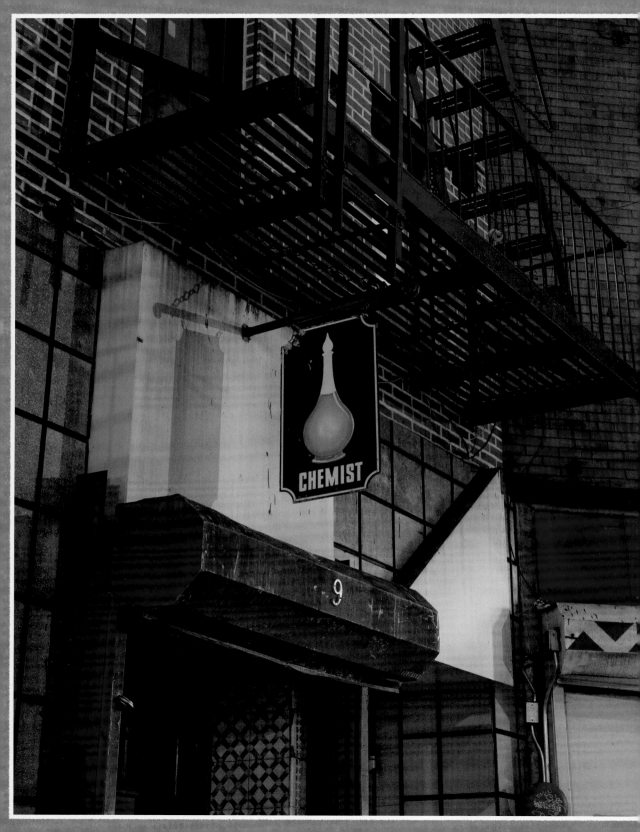

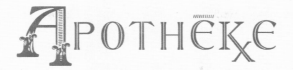

# APOTHEKE

## MODERN
## MEDICINAL
## COCKTAILS

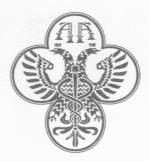

# CHRISTOPHER TIERNEY

### AND

# ERICA BROD

*with* Expert Insights *from* Apotheke Mixology Director
NICOLAS O'CONNOR

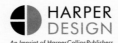

HARPER
DESIGN

An Imprint of HarperCollins Publishers

HarperCollins books may be purchased for educational, business, or
sales promotional use. For information please email the Special Markets
Department at SPsales@harpercollins.com.

First published in 2020 by
Harper Design
*An Imprint* of HarperCollins*Publishers*
195 Broadway
New York, NY 10007
Tel: (212) 207-7000
Fax: (855) 746-6023
harperdesign@harpercollins.com
www.hc.com

Distributed throughout the world by
HarperCollins*Publishers*
195 Broadway
New York, NY 10007

ISBN 978-0-06-299524-7

Library of Congress Control Number: 2020034263

*Book design by* Raphael Geroni

Printed in Canada

Second Printing, 2022

---

PAGE 2: The Apotheke NYC entrance is marked by subtle signage hinting at our apothecary roots.
PAGE 6: Austria-Hungary's coat of arms was the inspiration for Apotheke's brand icon.

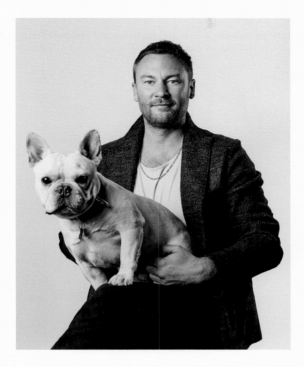

*May your spirit be free and flow*
*with the same mountains of love and*
*light you brought into the world.*

## CHRISTOPHER TIERNEY

### 1980-2022

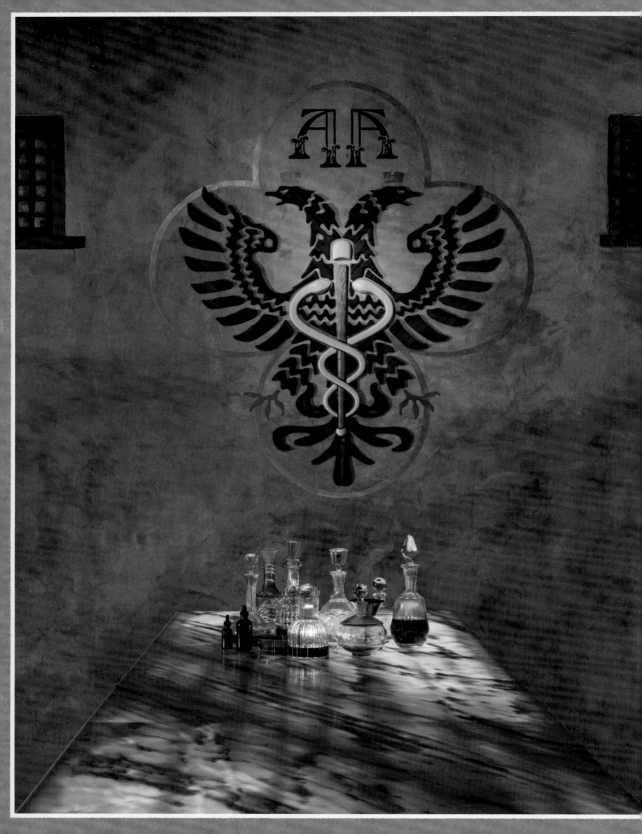

# CONTENTS

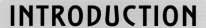

# INTRODUCTION

**F**OR MORE THAN A DECADE, WE AT APOTHEKE HAVE BEEN testing, tasting, creating, and collaborating; mixing chemistry with artistry; blending creativity with craft to offer our patrons excellence in the form of a cocktail. This book tells the story of Apotheke—old-world apothecary roots utilizing modern medicinal mixology. Born on the quiet streets of the Bloody Angle in Manhattan's Chinatown, Apotheke is now a bustling brand and one of the most notorious cocktail bars in New York City and beyond. An award-winning LA location opened in January 2018, and a second Manhattan location is in the works.

Inspired by the rise of the apothecary in Europe and the artistic influence of absinthe dens in nineteenth-century Paris, Apotheke is the first of its kind. Upon discovering the unmarked entrance on a desolate alley-like street, one walks through a heavy solid oak door into an opulent, antique interior. At Apotheke, our medicinal approach to the art of mixology offers a truly authentic experience. Patrons indulge in a spectrum of specialty cocktails infused with exotic herbs, fruits, and functional botanicals. The thirty-foot, glowing marble bar illuminates the cocktail chemistry and award-winning aesthetic. In a production where the muddler has become the modern-day mortar and pestle, Apotheke is much more than a bar; it is a cocktail

apothecary—elevating our patrons' experience through modern science flair and innovative flavor profiles using healing, natural ingredients.

Apotheke's unexpected and unassuming location has made it a sought-after destination and an immersive escape from the city. The 200-year-old wooden door and red velvet curtains are a portal into hypnotic, vintage luxury. The interior is a composition to a prolific past, a nod to 1800s Parisian apothecaries with an air of opium-den secrecy. Sumptuous and surreal, the experience defies and titillates the senses. Apotheke is an ode to the complex botanicals, elixirs, and herbs that have been used in remedies throughout time. We take an appreciative bow to the failed experiment of Prohibition, which legally codified alcohol as medicine and is forever romanticized in our collective consciousness.

Since opening in the fall of 2008, Apotheke has gained a global following of dedicated clientele and celebrity fans. The enduring popularity stems from its ability—especially notable in the Manhattan craft cocktail scene—to provide a multisensory experience with both style and substance. The mixologists, fitted in lab coats, take their craft seriously, pouring their energy and creativity into carefully selected glasses. They experiment behind the glowing marble platform with exotic, local herbs, botanicals, and tinctures—as ancient herbalists and apothecaries have done for thousands of years—until the perfect combination of science, art, taste, and balance harmonizes into a prodigious cocktail. Our Formula cocktails are divided into six sections based on function and ingredients: "Health & Beauty," "Aphrodisiacs," "Stress Relievers," "Stimulants," "Painkillers," and "Euphorics."

*Apotheke: Modern Medicinal Cocktails* equips you with all you need to bring your kitchen and bar together. We've selected fifty of our favorite proprietary recipes from both our New York City and Los Angeles locations. It is meant to be fun and informative with a dash of seriousness, and aimed to send you down the rabbit hole of medicinal mixology: crafting delicious drinks with love and quality ingredients. We invite you to experience firsthand the repertoire that took Apotheke from an experiment to an institution.

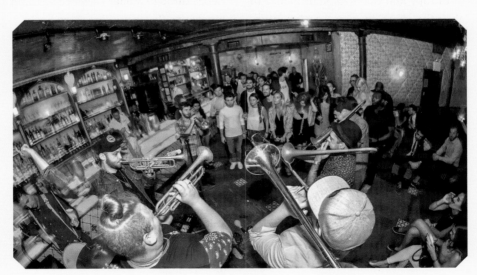

High & Mighty Brass Band has been making our Tuesday nights special for years, bringing high energy and good vibes as the full brass band pumps out pulsating beats that meld old-school funk with modern hip hop.

# A NEW CONCEPT FLICKERS TO LIFE

**A**POTHEKE IS NEW YORK CITY'S ORIGINAL COCKTAIL apothecary. We got our start nestled in the heart of Manhattan's historic China-town, on a tiny bent street with a violent history involving Chinese gang warfare, underground tunnels, opium dens, and hatchet murders. So infamous is Doyers Street that in the early 1900s, it earned the nickname "The Bloody Angle" for having more people die violently at this intersection than any other intersection in the country. At a time when Chinatown was known only for Chinese restaurants, massage parlors, and herb shops, Apotheke signed an atypical lease at the apex of the angle.

Chinatown is a jarring combination, at once unwaveringly local and intensely touristy. The Chinese community has successfully resisted pressures to alter the face of its neighborhood and bring in major new developments, so the enclave feels more like China than downtown Manhattan. Signage is mostly in Chinese, leaving one to communicate with hand signals to the butchers and fishmongers. The one thing it has in common with the rest of Manhattan is the density of people rushing through the streets.

During the day, people from all over the world converge in this slice of the city. Busy Canal Street and the surrounding streets are lined with shops selling kitschy New York souvenirs, and little plastic pools teem with battery-powered swimming frogs. There's the occasional caricature artist on the street and the man selling bubble machines, relentlessly shooting shiny orbs onto the sidewalk. Exotic fruit and vegetable stands color the sidewalk. At dawn, parks are packed with elderly people practicing tai chi to traditional Chinese music.

On Doyers Street, cooks chain-smoke on stoops and cracking vinyl chairs under the dizzying swirl of barber poles, observing the excited tourists taking photo-graphs. Visitors may catch a spontaneous

*Doyers Street is named after Hendrik Doyer, a Dutch immigrant who arrived in the 1700s. He ran a distillery where the post office currently stands, and the street began as a cobblestoned horse cart path to serve the distillery.*

performance by the street's resident martial arts demonstrator: an elderly Chinese man often practices in the middle of the street, sometimes shirtless, sometimes taking a break, meticulously eating his lunch from a Styrofoam container.

Doyers resembles an alley more than a street, and it is one of the very few with an L shape in Manhattan. A mere 200 feet long, Doyers Street's sharp angle gives it a unique perspective. It is said that superstition is responsible for the street's shape, as it was laid in this shape because "straight-flying ghosts" wouldn't be able to take the turn. It is impossible to see the end of the street from either the Pell Street side or the Bowery/Chatham Square/Division Street side. (This provided an advantageous escape for Tong members post-massacre and -ambush.) The tiny street has a reputation that far exceeds its size, with throngs of tourists visiting daily to hear about its weighted history and photograph the attractions.

Sometimes two different tour group companies are on the street at the same time, the guides competing for who can be the loudest. They regale their groups with violent stories of the Tong Wars and the mystique of former opium dens and underground tunnels. They usually butcher the pronunciation of Apotheke (it's pronounced *Ap-o-teck*), as is true of many new and returning patrons. However, this has somehow added to the attractive mystique of the brand. (*Apotheke* is German for "pharmacy.")

At night, Doyers Street is quiet. It's lit from above by a pale yellow glow emitted from Chinese-style streetlamps and bright fluorescent bulbs filtered through faded storefront signs. The feeling is part eerie and part romantic. Turning onto Doyers from Pell or Bowery for the first time, one may think they've stumbled upon a Macau marketplace circa 1950.

Amidst this is a destination one would least expect to be here: cocktail apothecary meets speakeasy lounge, where a seasoned craft cocktail scene anchors the atmosphere. The mood is saturated in bespoke glamour and bygone eras. It usually takes first-time patrons a few laps up and down Doyers Street to find the dimly lit, old European oak door, beautiful and out of place; the only clue is a small "Chemist" plaque protruding from the facade above the door.

The cozy, sleek atmosphere of Apotheke is a surreal contrast to the neighborhood outside. The heavy wooden door closes and seals out the juxtaposed exterior. It's time to enter the Apotheke experience.

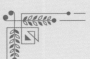 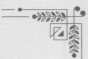

# THE BLOODY ANGLE AND THE NEW YORK TONG WARS

**T**HE SORDID PAST OF OUR DOYERS STREET HOME IS RIFE with murder, mayhem, hatchet men, underground escape tunnels, assassins, and opium dens.

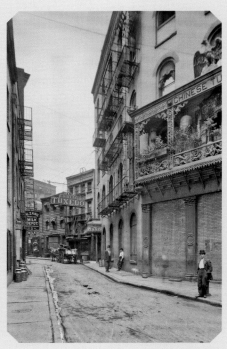

Chinese immigrants organized three types of mutual aid societies upon arriving in the United States. Tong, which means "chamber," is the third category, consisting of sworn brotherhoods, with no geographic or family requirements. The Hip Sing Tong and the On Leong Tong became fierce rivals, fighting over gambling, prostitution, opium, and pride.

The New York Tong Wars raged for three decades in Chinatown, with most of the battles taking place on Pell Street, Mott Street, and Doyers Street.

## Timeline

- 1900: The murder of Hip Sing member Lung Kin on Pell Street launches the First Tong War.
- 1905: Previously considered neutral ground by the tongs, four On Leong members are murdered at the Chinese Theater during a play. As revenge, the On Leongs pin down Hip Sing laundryman Hop Lee on his ironing board, hit him repeatedly with a meat cleaver, and hack off his nose.

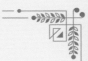

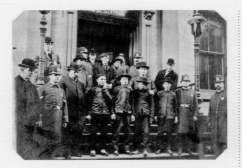

🖝 **1933:** Doyers Street is the site of the last person to die in the Tong Wars.

🖝 **1934:** The end of the wars.

🖝 **2008:** Apotheke opens for business on Doyers Street.

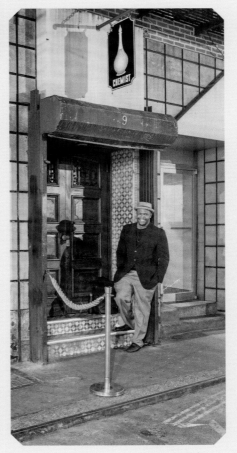

🖝 **1909:** The murder of Bow Kum launches the Second Tong War. Bow Kum, wife of an On Leong Tong member, was formerly enslaved by a Four Brothers man who was suspected in her murder. The Four Brothers, a clan society made up of four Chinese families, becomes enemy number one for the On Leongs.

🖝 **1910:** Doyers Street is first referred to as the Bloody Angle of Chinatown.

🖝 **1912:** The Third Tong War, over the opium trade, begins.

🖝 **1924:** The Hip Sings allow Chin Jack Lem to switch sides, leading to the Fourth Tong War. He had been high up in the On Leong ranks in Chicago, but the tong ousted him. This drove him into the arms of the Hip Sing, claiming he could bring other defectors. The revenge attacks and tensions over loyalties spread to tongs in other cities.

OPPOSITE: Snakelike Doyers Street, sometimes called "Murder Alley" during the New York Tong Wars, is pictured from the Bowery in 1901. • TOP: Members of the rival secret societies Hip Sing Tong, led by the death-defying Mock Duck, and On Leong Tong, ruled by Tammany Hall–connected Tom Lee, stand outside a police station after their arrests for the Pell Street Chinese New Year ambush in 1906. • BOTTOM: Lamont Goings stands at six feet two inches and has a deep, gravelly voice. His stature may make people think twice about causing trouble, but he's a big teddy bear. Lamont has helmed as doorman for Apotheke NYC since 2009.

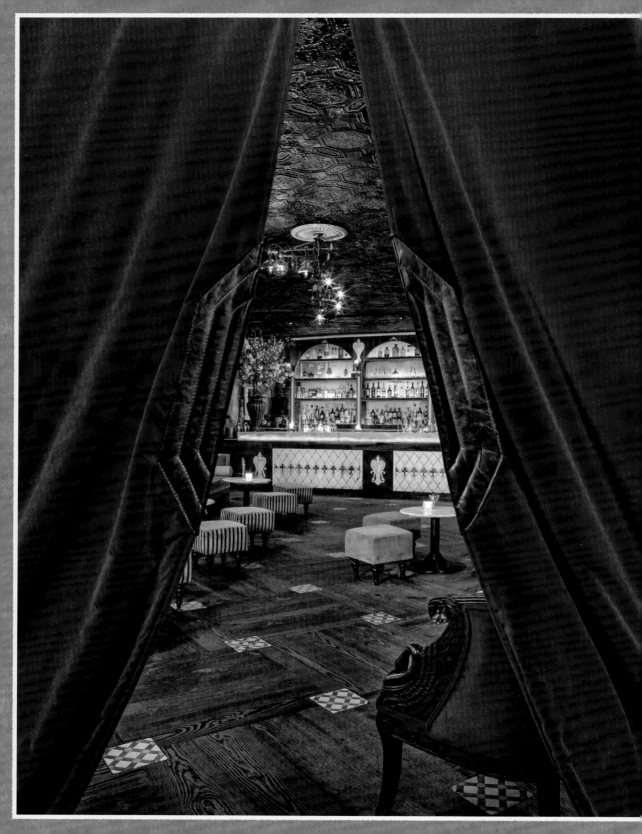

# APOTHEKE'S INTERIOR

*by Founder and Designer*
CHRISTOPHER TIERNEY

**A**S AN ARTIST-ENTREPRENEUR AND EXPLORER AT HEART, my appreciation and connection to the natural world has always been the effervescent part of my spirit and inspiration. With every design project, there is a moment when I experience an indescribable exhilaration, when I lock on to the core concept and allow the laws of attraction to drive the creative process. I find the universe can be quite generous in this moment; it's when I feel most alive.

*For Apotheke, the concept was simple but infinitely robust:*

A VINTAGE APOTHECARY
AND ITS TREASURE CHEST OF INSPIRATION.

OPPOSITE: Enter the cocktail apothecary, tucked away behind the red velvet curtains.
FOLLOWING SPREAD: The thirty-foot bar is made of a rare marble from a quarry in Portugal.

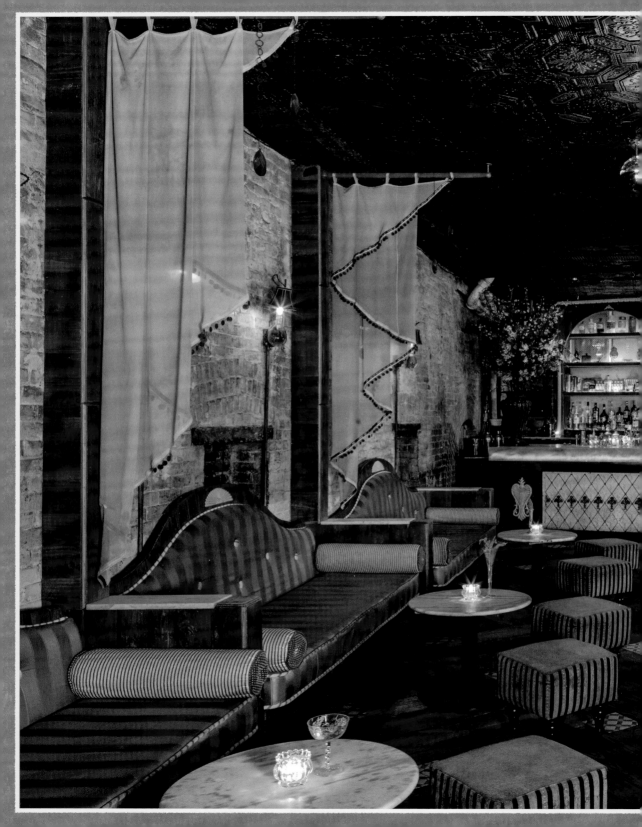

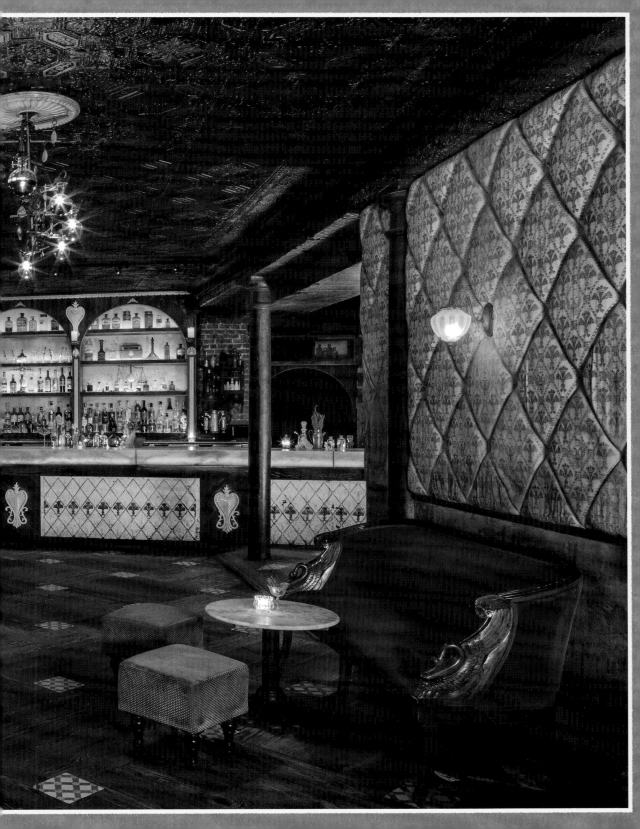

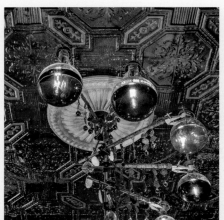

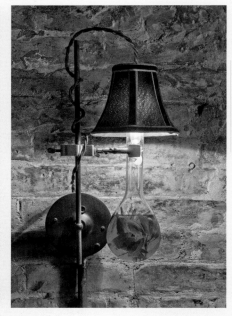

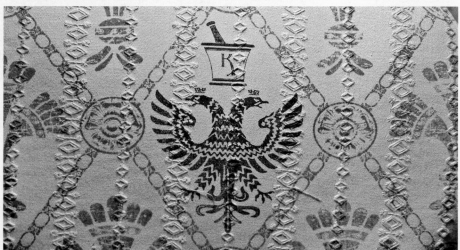

CLOCKWISE FROM TOP LEFT: From the reclaimed pine floors with inlaid tiles to discovering and restoring the original tin ceiling, as seen illuminated by our beaker chandelier centerpiece, it was a labor of love. ⬩ Old-school apothecary show globe meets modern chemistry fusion in our customized light fixtures with colored liquid and suspended botanicals illuminated in glass chemistry vessels. ⬩ The fabric wall design contains one of an apothecary's go-to tools: the mortar and pestle. ⬩ OPPOSITE: The original NYC wall sculpture and brand icon. FOLLOWING SPREAD: An array of bottles in the front window harkens back to apothecaries of the past.

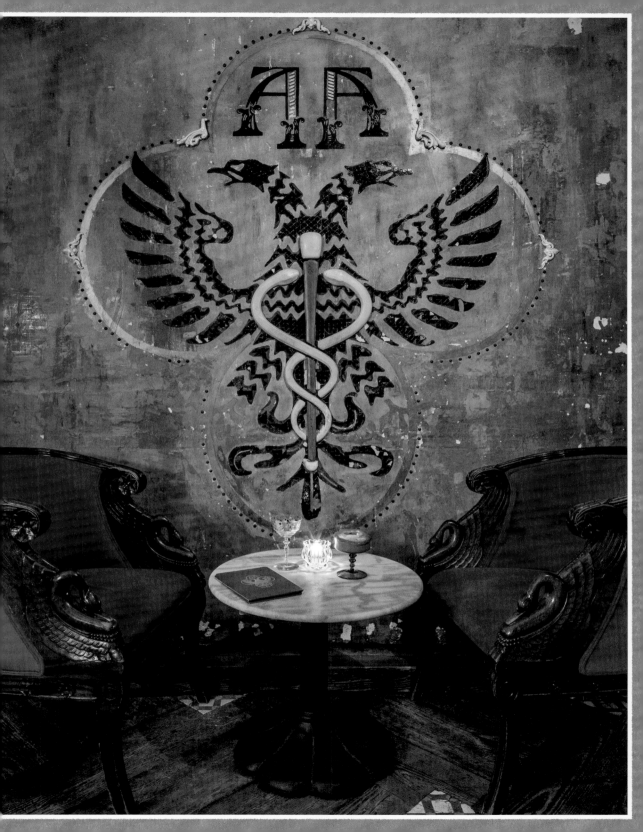

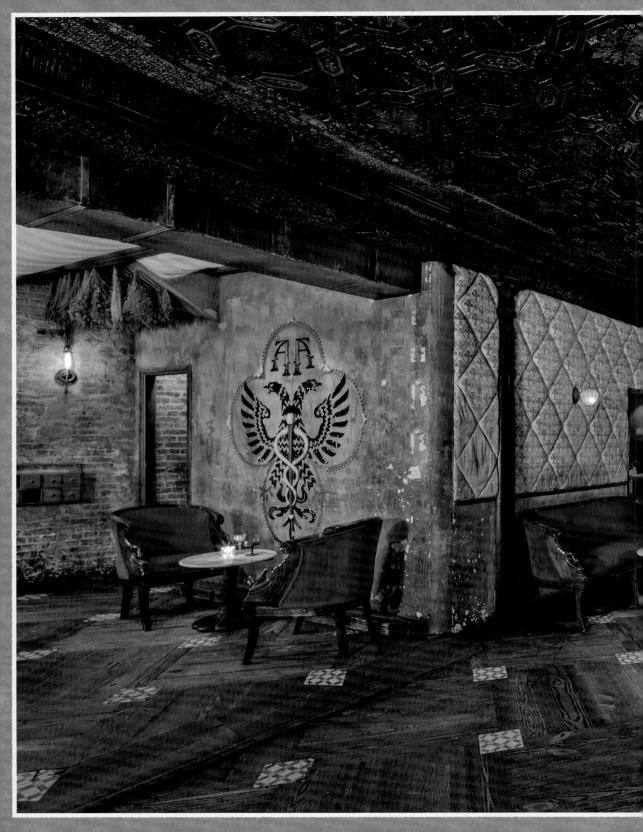

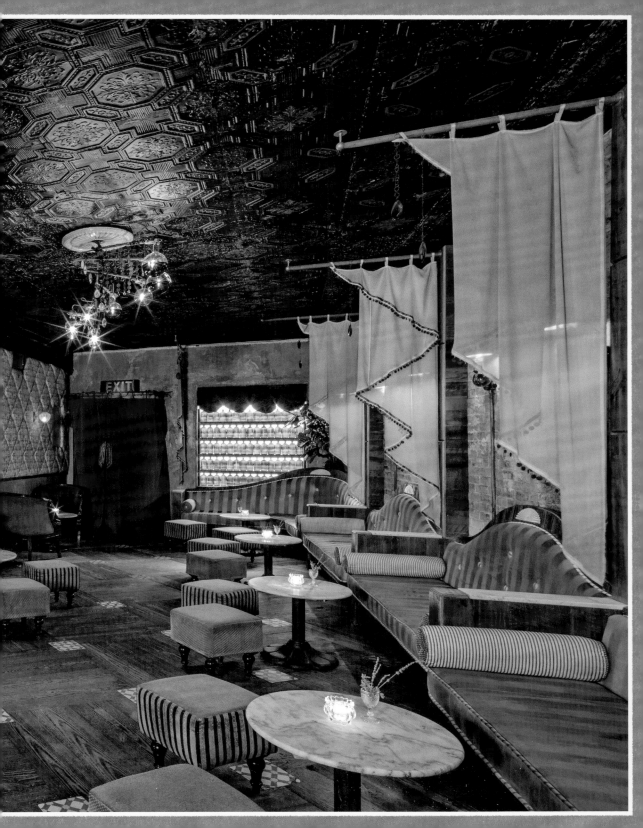

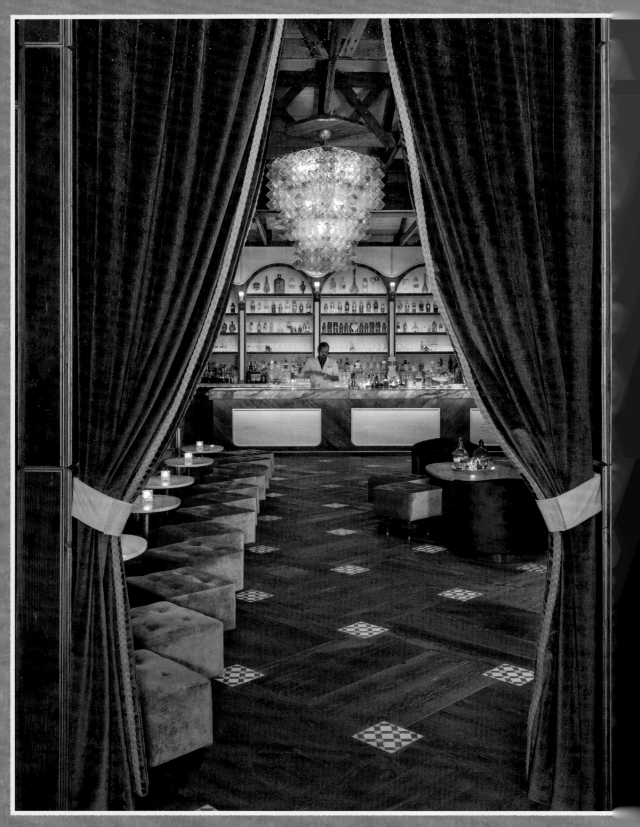

# APOTHEKE WEST COAST

## *Apotheke Los Angeles*

**A**S WE CELEBRATED OUR TEN-YEAR ANNIVERSARY IN NEW York City, we opened Apotheke on the West Coast in January 2018. As with the East Coast location, tucked away on a remote street, Apotheke Los Angeles sits in the shadow of a bridge next to the Los Angeles River. It is another destination experience, also located in Chinatown, in the industrial noodle-packing district. The interior is akin to Apotheke New York City—including the glowing marble bar—with additional desirable attributes thanks to LA's warm weather. It has an outdoor patio constructed from reclaimed ceiling joists and an adjacent herb garden to source ingredients year-round. The marble bar continues outside under a canvas cabana flanked with oversized pots spilling over with herbs and botanicals.

Apotheke LA launched innovative new creations tailored for the West Coast lifestyle, including spirit-free wellness tonics. The tonics are composed of medicinal herbs and organic botanicals. Each is engineered from a base that is made from Apotheke's proprietary tea blends, specifically designed to deliver different health functions.

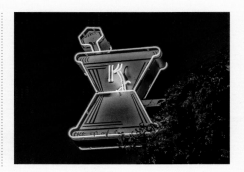

OPPOSITE: We kept the rich velvet material for LA's entryway but switched up the color, opting for blue instead of NYC's sumptuous red. • ABOVE: The symbol for an Apothecary glows above the Apotheke LA entrance in Chinatown. • FOLLOWING SPREAD: The LA bar is made from the same imported marble as the one in NYC.

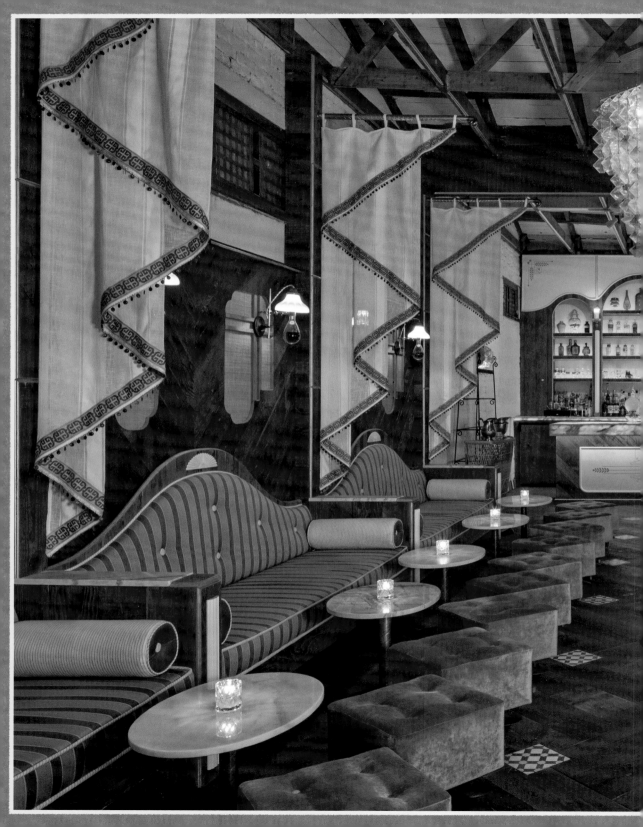

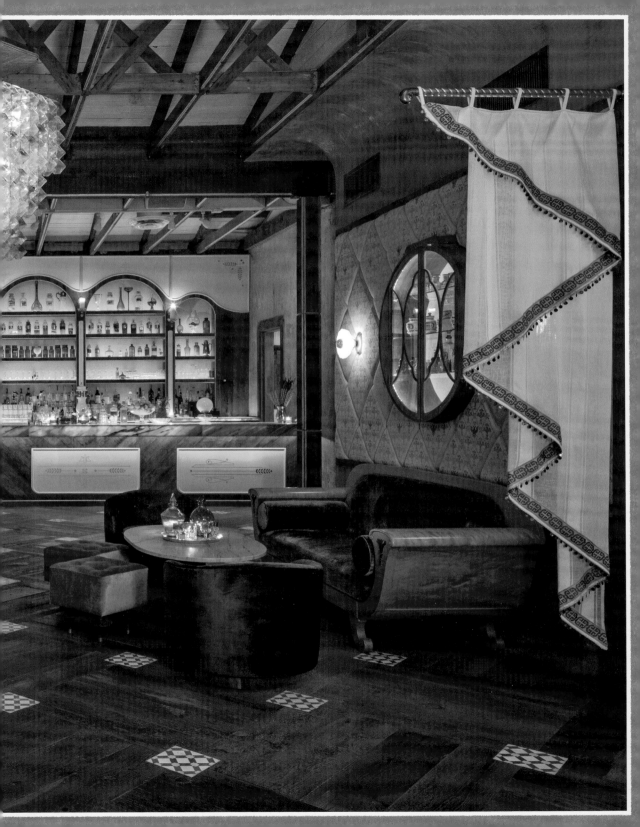

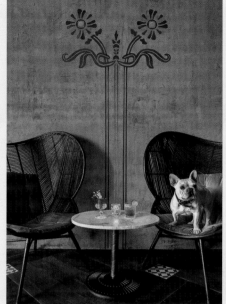
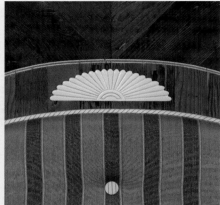
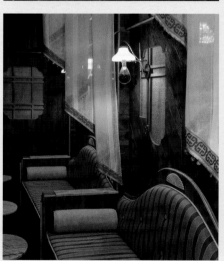
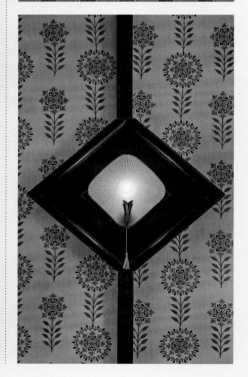

CLOCKWISE FROM TOP LEFT: Christopher's pup patiently poses in front of a hand-painted mural at Apotheke LA. • Porcelain appliqué details the Apotheke LA seating. • Apotheke LA sconce against an embroidered plant-adorned fabric wall. • With the practice gained by doing the same in NYC, we built the banquettes and ottomans by hand. • OPPOSITE: Apotheke Mixology Director Nicolas O'Connor pours with a smile at the outside bar. • FOLLOWING SPREAD: The garden patio takes advantage of LA's lovely weather.

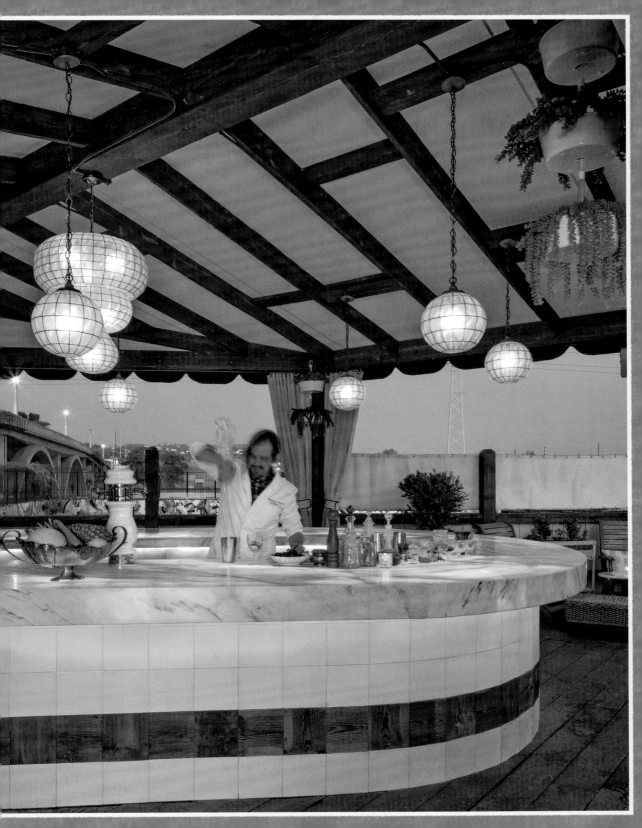

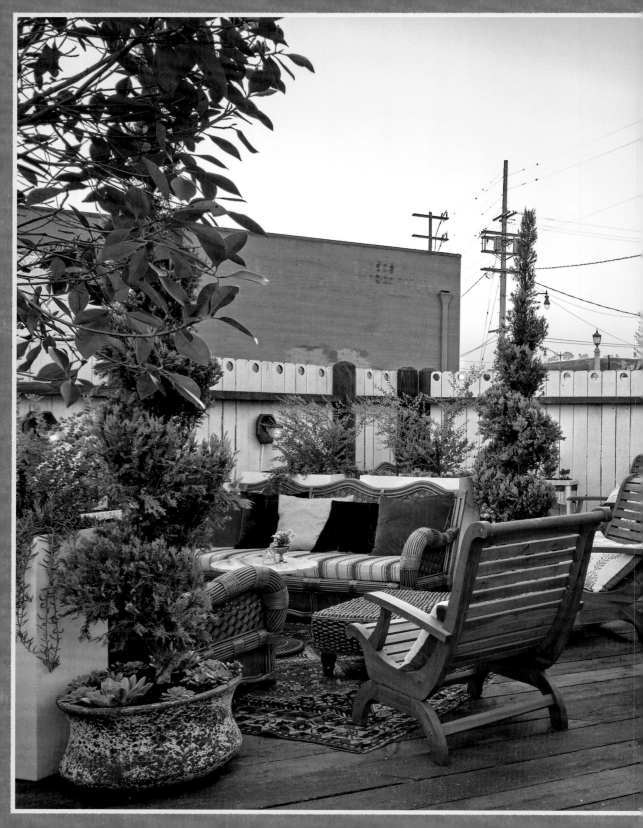

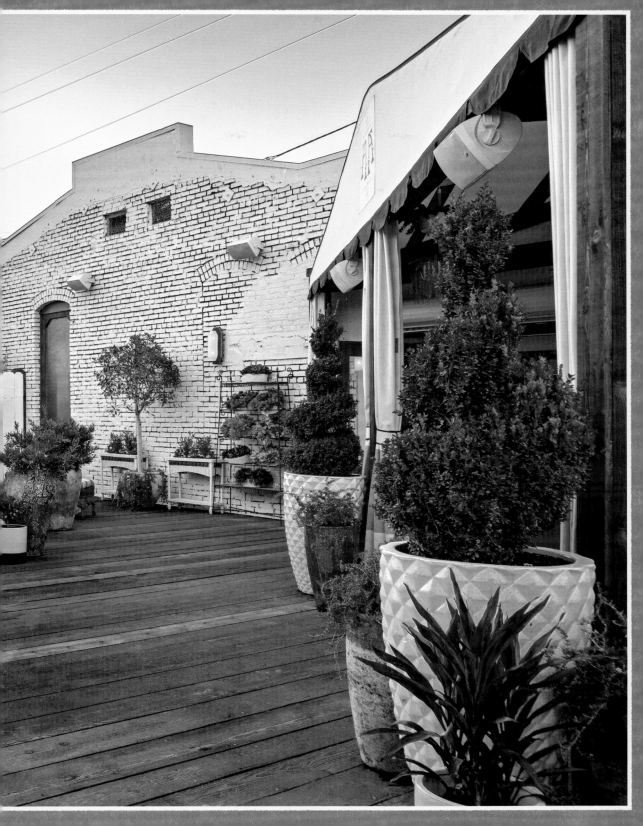

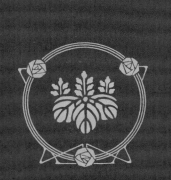

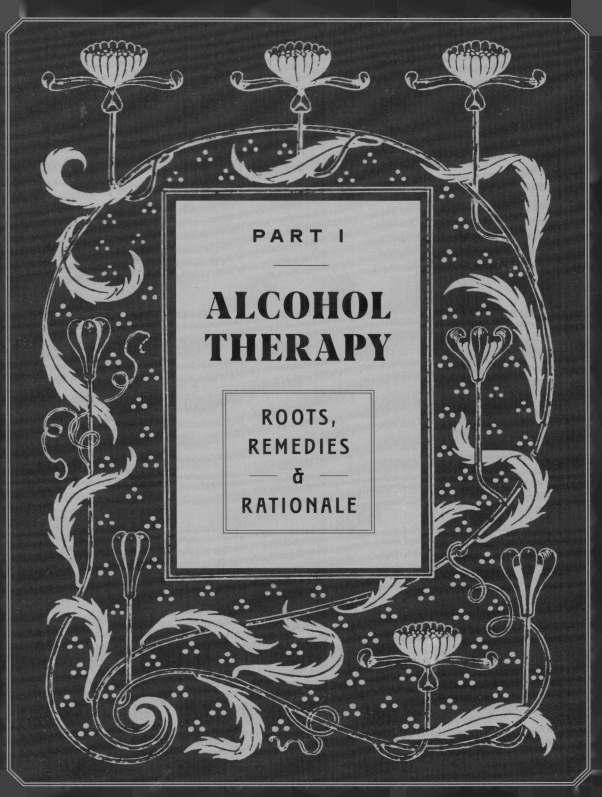

# PART I

## ALCOHOL THERAPY

### ROOTS, REMEDIES & RATIONALE

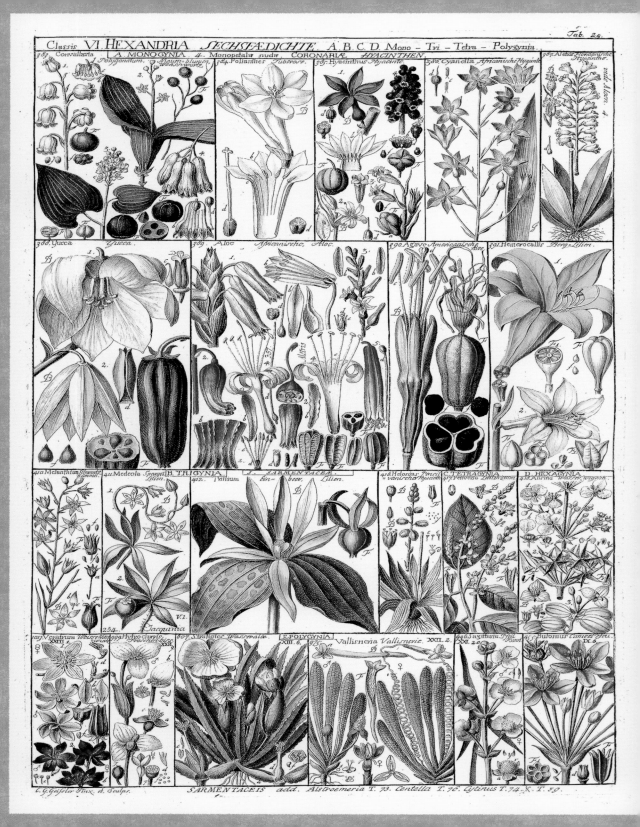

Tab. 25.

Classis VI. HEXANDRIA SECHSFAEDICHTE. A.B.C.D. Mono - Tri - Tetra - Polygynia.

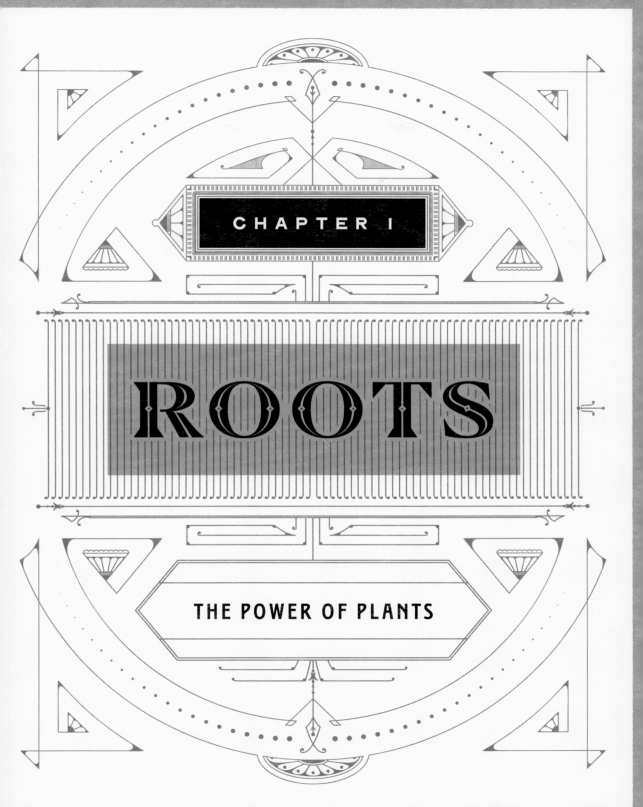

CHAPTER I

ROOTS

THE POWER OF PLANTS

*Nature is the chief physician.*

—Dr. Elisha Smith, *The Botanic Physician* (1830)

**P**LANTS HAVE BEEN USED MEDICINALLY BY ALL CULTURES, from the beginning of our time on the planet to the present. They are a universal thread and shared experience connecting all humans throughout time, from the farthest corners of the globe.

There are approximately 380,000 identified plant species across the globe, with an average of 2,000 new species discovered annually. It is estimated that only 10 percent of these species have been examined for pharmacological use. In the early 2000s, there were around 50,000 medicinal plants in use around the world.

The pharmaceutical industry used vascular plants in nearly all of its research until the 1950s. With the discovery of antibiotics and synthetic drugs, scientists became enamored with the idea that man-made chemicals could be a cure for everything. It was like a kid with a shiny new toy that irresistibly pulls him away from his old standby toys. Antibiotics were,

of course, revolutionary. But the exclusive focus on man-made chemicals has, over time, rendered traditional medicine and local healing expertise invisible and dismissed. Long before the 1928 discovery of penicillin, Central American Indian and Chinese healers had been successfully using fermented soybean curd for skin infections, and voodoo practitioners recommended moldy bread for syphilis sufferers. They didn't know why these things worked, but they knew that they did.

Human health proved to be a trickier beast to tame—and diseases more complex, intractable, and variable from person to person—than pharmaceutical companies assumed. Some synthetic drugs have

Aesculapius, the Greek god of medicine pictured on the left of this 1864 apothecary card, wields his one-serpent staff—the traditional symbol of medicine—accompanied by Hebe, the Greek goddess of youth.

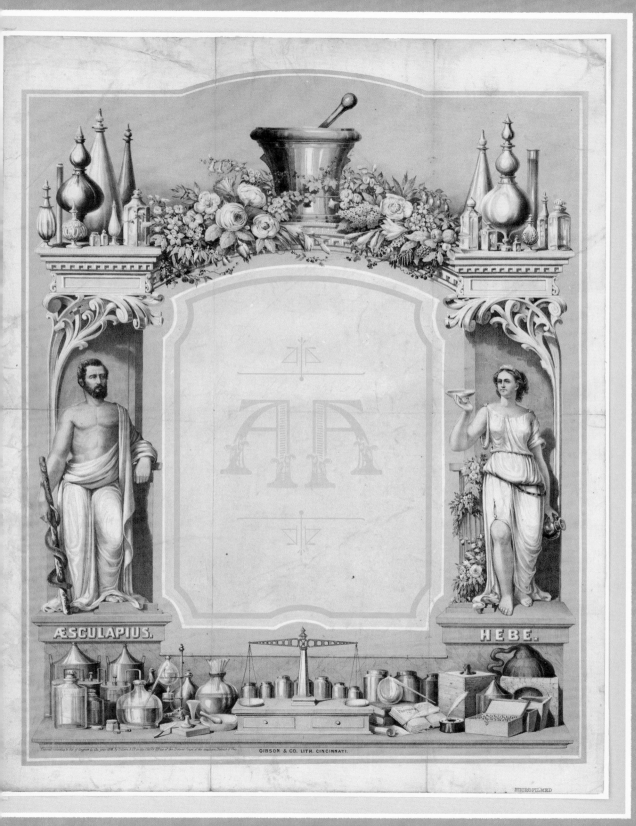

AESCULAPIUS.

HEBE.

GIBSON & CO. LITH. CINCINNATI.

proven to decline in efficacy with use, and many have a host of contraindications. They didn't produce the prolific cures that had been (naively) expected of them. These disappointing results brought companies full circle, and they again started to seek out herbal medicines around the world. Plants have evolved alongside humans. As such, their interactions with human cells are multifaceted, and they have a large array of beneficial effects that go to work preventing, fighting, and protecting against disease in the human body. You just can't replace that biodynamic interaction. We are part of nature; it seems a given that nature would thus provide us with human-friendly remedies.

## Pharmaceutical Applications of Nature

- The drug aspidium is made from the rhizome and stipes of the fern *Dryopteris marginalis*.
- Aspirin's natural base, willow bark, has been used as a remedy for thousands of years.
- The 1960 discovery of the wild rosy periwinkle in Madagascar led to the production of the chemotherapy drugs vincristine and vinblastine. The drugs lowered childhood leukemia mortalities and boosted remission rates for Hodgkin's disease patients.
- Yams proved useful for contraceptive medications. In the late 1940s, a chemist synthesized progestin from the root of the Mexican wild yam, and shortly thereafter, in 1950, an oral contraceptive pill, which uses synthetic progestin, was produced.
- In 2002, a Danish start-up company, MediMush, launched, supplying medicinal mushroom ingredients to the pharmaceutical industry. Mushrooms are popular immune-system boosters, and they contain compounds that can treat cancer. MediMush pioneered the first oral form of the polysaccharide lentinan from shiitake mushrooms.
- Artemisinin, an effective antimalarial compound, is derived from sweet wormwood, or *qinghao*. It was identified by studying traditional Chinese medicine, which has used qinghao for thousands of years to treat malaria.

Our forebears had to rely on trial and error (sometimes fatal), instinct, and oral tradition in choosing their plant remedies. Scientists have identified several plant compounds that impact our physiological well-being, including phytochemicals, polyphenols, tannins, ellagic acid, anthocyanins, and more. They recognized that many of plants' medicinal qualities come from secondary metabolites—meaning that plants don't need them to survive; they have developed them as a sophisticated way of interacting with their environment and maintaining resilience in it (including resilience against animals that eat them, like us). Plants have a mysterious power to work on our bodies and minds that the modern medical community is still trying to decipher and map out.

This is an exciting time for plant-based medicine. The 2000s have been characterized by a rejection of the industrial and artificial. People want craft, quality, and local. Our society is returning to our roots. More and more people are turning to plants and what is referred to as "folk" or "traditional" medicine, which is largely the result of indigenous cultures accumulating and transmitting knowledge from

generation to generation. The limitations of synthetic drugs have led to renewed attention to plants and their complex chemical constituents. Mainstream science is finally catching on, and researchers are exploring the different biochemical pathways of medicinal plants, their active compounds, the best traditional and modern ways of extracting bioactive material, and ensuring they're safe in clinical trials. The numbers are promising: medicinal plant research publications have tripled in the past decade, from 4,686 in 2008 to 14,884 in 2018.

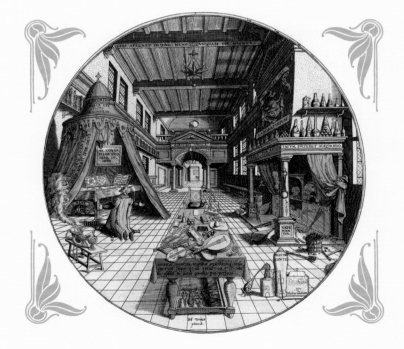

Alchemists intertwined magic with science in their drive to understand and purify matter, nature, and the human body, as captured in "Alchemist's Laboratory" from Heinrich Khunrath's famous *Amphitheatrum Sapientiae Aeternae* ("Amphitheater of Eternal Wisdom"), 1595.

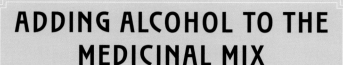

# ADDING ALCOHOL TO THE MEDICINAL MIX

*It is hard to think of an illness, disease, or physical pathology that has not, at some time, been treated by some form of alcohol. It has been credited with ridding the body of worms and cancer, aiding digestion, fighting heart disease, and turning back old age and extending life itself.*

—ROD PHILLIPS, *Alcohol: A History* (2014)

**ALL ALCOHOL COMES FROM PLANTS. PLANTS TAKE IN** sunshine and carbon dioxide, producing sugar and emitting oxygen. Single-celled yeasts eat sugar and produce ethanol and carbon dioxide as waste products in a process called fermentation. Ethanol excretion is a way for yeasts to keep competing microbes at bay—they're toxic to them. We benefit from this antimicrobial effect when we drink alcohol.

Once the concentration of alcohol reaches 15 percent, however, the yeasts die—they have sealed their own fate. To make alcohol stronger than 15 percent alcohol by volume (ABV), we need to turn to distillation. Distillation takes advantage of the fact that alcohol has a lower boiling point than water. Heat is applied so that the mixture boils off the alcohol, but not the water, and the alcohol is then cooled and condensed into a collecting container. The resulting liquid is a higher proof spirit.

Depicted on the title page of Oswald Croll's *Basilica Chymica* (1609), with its infamous mix of enigmatic mysticism and groundbreaking scientific experimentation, alchemy set the stage for medicinal spirits. Some alchemists believed that they discovered the universal remedy in distilled alcohol.

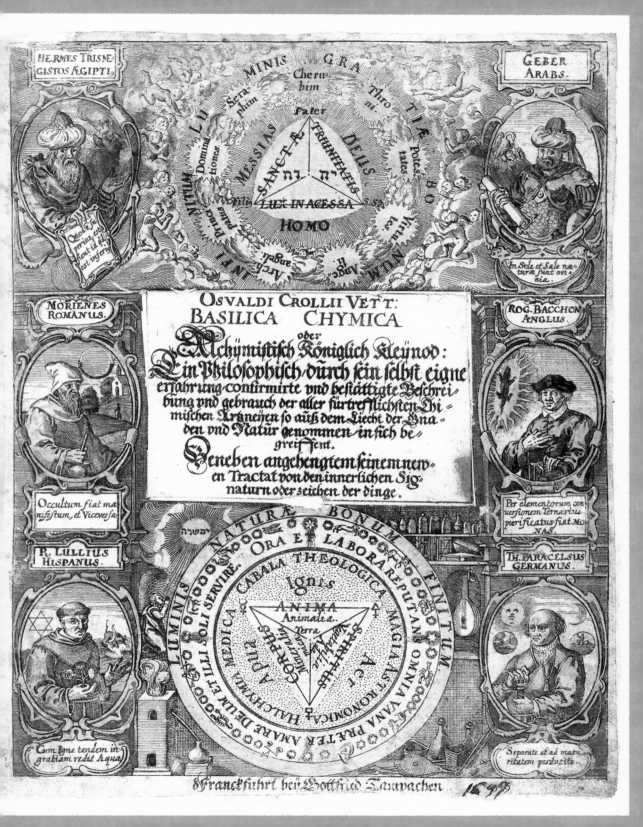

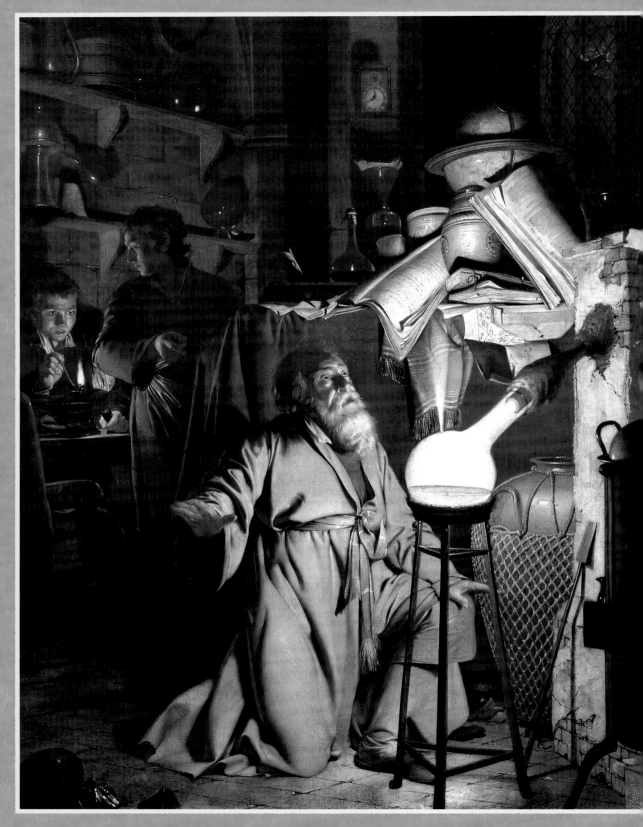

# HAPPY ACCIDENTS + ALCHEMICAL EXPERIMENTATION = SPIRITS

**S**PIRITS CAN TRACE THEIR HERITAGE TO THE UNIQUE relationship between yeast, plants, water, heat, and human ingenuity.

While ancient cultures stumbled upon the happy accident of fermentation that allowed them to drink wine, beer, and mead, distilling stronger alcohol required some intervention. It's believed that Arabs perfected distillation techniques in pursuit of essential oils and perfumes, and their technology spread to Europe. Alcohol historians trace the first production of spirits to around 1150 CE. However, some historians have provided evidence of even earlier distillation practices in India and China, with the first liquor creation variously attributed to Arab alchemists or Italian monks.

Egyptians were early experimenters with the alembic still, now called the pot still. In an alembic still design, a tube connects two long-necked vessels. When using an alembic still, distillers have to clean everything each time, which limits production. In 1831, the column still was invented, which gave distillers some advantages and efficiencies. The column still is also called the continuous still for a good reason: it allows distillers to keep on distilling, without needing to stop and clean everything in between runs. It's a 24-7 world, and the column still brings that to the distillation process.

Alchemy has long captured the imagination—and rebuke—of society. Shrouded in secrecy, alchemy was one of chemistry's predecessors, and its adherents were focused on transformation. They sought to create gold, an elixir of life-granting immortality, the philosopher's stone, medical cures, and more. Alchemists were among the pioneers of distillation, as they believed it could extract the

Often (understandably) shortened to *The Alchymist*, the full title of Joseph Wright's 1771 painting is *The Alchymist, in Search of the Philosopher's Stone, discovers Phosphorus, and prays for the successful conclusion of his operation, as was the custom of the ancient chymical astrologers.*

quintessence—the underlying force—of all things. Their quest for an elixir of life paved the way for the first distilled spirits.

All spirits are created by fermenting and distilling botanical ingredients. After distillation, water is added before bottling to bring the spirit down to the desired alcohol percentage.

The first distilled spirits in Europe were called *aqua vitae* or *eau de vie*, the "water of life," and they were distilled from materials that were readily available: first wines, then fruits and grains. Apothecaries and monasteries were the main purveyors of alcohol for several centuries, prescribing it as medicinal cordials and general healing tonics. This nomenclature demonstrates the swift attribution of healing properties to the new class of higher proof alcohol; by the thirteenth century, aqua vitae was receiving considerable attention for its medicinal potential. Distilled liquors became more widespread in the fifteenth and sixteenth centuries as they moved beyond the apothecary into the recreational realm. However, the belief that spirits held medicinal value, and their use in medicines, persisted into the nineteenth century and beyond. Alcohol-based curatives took an interesting turn during Prohibition. Alcohol prescribed for medicinal use was deemed legal, so pharmacists started dispensing alcohol prescriptions.

Plants were our first medicines; it is their mystical healing nature that has allowed humans to survive and thrive.

We must also be eternally grateful to plants for giving us one of the most enduring relationships we have: alcohol. Dating back to the earliest practices of medicine in ancient cultures, alcohol has been used as a therapeutic remedy and a way of unleashing the curative properties of plants.

At this time, *when* humans had their earliest experiences with alcohol is a moving target; so far, evidence from pottery jars shows that the earliest deliberate concoction of a mixed alcoholic drink was in Neolithic Jiahu, China, around 7000 BCE. In his landmark analysis in the early 2000s, biomolecular archaeologist Patrick McGovern confirmed that the jars contained a fermented drink made of rice, fruit (grapes and/or hawthorn berries), and honey. Humans probably consumed alcohol before 7000 BCE, but they might have stored the alcohol in vessels that would disintegrate, taking any evidence with them. Early alcohol remnants in China and the Middle East, notably, contain plant material that was not utilized in the making of the alcohol; this would indicate that the botanicals were added as flavor, medicine, or both.

McGovern's sophisticated biomolecular archaeology uncovered another breakthrough in ancient Egyptian wine vessels. His chemical analysis demonstrated that as far back as 3150 BCE, Egyptians were mixing herbs into their wine. We also know from ancient Egyptian papyrus medical scrolls that they combined coriander, flax, dates, and bryony with beer and drank it as a stomach remedy. This is some of the earliest and strongest evidence to date that they were using alcohol and botanicals medicinally.

Wine and beer, whether alone or mixed with medicinal barks, roots, spices, and seeds, were common remedies. Hippocrates, the father of modern medicine, used alcohol-based herbal remedies, including wine infused with herbs, for intestinal worms in 400 BCE. Pliny the Elder recommended wine as a digestive aid. Wormwood-infused wine was another common remedy in early medicine for digestive issues.

And Europeans weren't the only ancient cultures that linked wine to health; the very first Chinese pharmaceutical writings highlighted wine's importance as a medicine, describing it as an antiseptic, anesthetic, and diuretic. We see echoes of the alchemists here too: wine showed up in the Taoist period's longevity elixirs.

By the early 1870s, alcohol was a common treatment for typhoid, typhus, and fevers. It was also used as an analgesic and sedative before and after surgeries, and it was given as a diuretic and appetite stimulant. Alcohol was prescribed frequently for therapeutic purposes until the 1920s.

## ALCOHOL AND BOTANICALS
### BRING OUT THE BEST

High-proof alcohol is a common vehicle for the therapeutic properties of botanicals. Liquor acts as a solvent and extracts the medicinal qualities of herbs and plants, including resins, alkaloids, glycosides, and volatile oils. Alcohol's chemical composition renders it particularly adept at penetrating cell membranes, as well as extracting carotenoid pigments and aroma molecules from cells. Not only is alcohol better suited for dissolving solids than water, it also preserves fresh ingredients by helping to prevent fermentation. Bitters and tinctures generally use the highest-proof alcohol possible to get the most out of their herbal constituents.

Apotheke's proprietary line of Bitters with Benefits™, APO, is the perfect modern example: expert-chosen botanical ingredients macerated in high-proof ethanol to create medicinal formulas that function both as wellness tinctures and cocktail flavorings (page 96).

# BENEFITS OF THE APOTHEKE COCKTAIL

**F**OR THOUSANDS OF YEARS, PHYSICIANS AND APOTHECARIES believed in the therapeutic effects of alcoholic drinks and prescribed them liberally. Apotheke's mission is to understand alcohol consumption as an inherent part of human culture and offer products that are conscious of health, wellness, and alcohol's relationship to medicinal function. We view our cocktails as a way to pair real nutrients with alcohol consumption; for example, drinking just one Tainted Love (page 107) packs the nutritional equivalent of several helpings of beets. Like any modern medicine or regulated substance, apothecary cocktails are designed to be treated with the same discipline—where specific doses are defined so a product can achieve its positive effect.

Decades of studies have found positive effects of moderate drinking, including protection from coronary heart disease and stroke. Alcohol reduces the cholesterol buildup on artery walls that contribute to heart attacks, and it thins the blood, decreases coronary inflammation, and prevents blood clots in the heart. A study in England found that moderate drinkers came down with half the number of colds as nondrinkers.

The ongoing 90+ Study, conducted by neurologists from the University of California at Irvine, finds that moderate drinkers live longer than those who drink no alcohol. Researchers from several university medical centers found lower risks of dementia among older adults who were light or moderate drinkers compared to nondrinkers.

In a study reported in the *Journal of the American College of Cardiology* in 2017, researchers used a dataset of 333,247 people

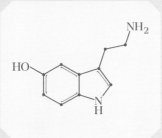

Drinking alcohol releases serotonin (the chemical structure shown here) and other key neurotransmitters, resulting in a warm, fuzzy feeling of well-being.

to look at alcohol use and mortality. They found that "compared with lifetime abstainers, those who were light or moderate alcohol consumers were at a reduced risk of mortality for all causes and cardiovascular disease (CVD). . . . Light and moderate alcohol intake might have a protective effect on all-cause and CVD-specific mortality in U.S. adults." The article also cites a meta-analysis that concluded that all alcoholic drinks in moderation were correlated with less heart disease risk, indicating that the benefit is due to ethanol, and not a compound specific to certain types of drinks.

The potentially life-giving effects apply to all types of alcohol. While we know that alcohol has a restorative effect, in and of itself, scientists are still trying to unravel the exact mechanisms. They know the *what*; they just want to find out the *how*.

This need to understand the underlying mechanisms is perhaps one of the reasons that plant-based remedies confound modern mainstream medicine so much. Cultures around the world have used herbs successfully for thousands of years. Even if they do not know the specific actions of each plant compound on human cells, they know the whole plant, and they know it works.

Digestifs, after-dinner drinks meant to soothe the stomach, have science to back them up: research shows that alcohol stimulates the secretion of digestive hormones. In the United States and Europe, bitters were prescribed for stomach and respiratory issues. Bitters are a natural extension of the mysterious, herb-laden liquors developed by monks and distillers.

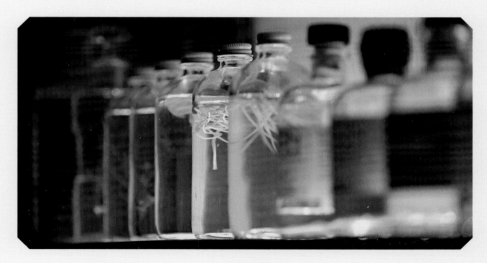

Alcohol and plants elevate each other like partners in a good marriage.

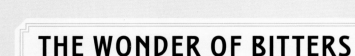

# THE WONDER OF BITTERS

**B**ITTERS ARE AROMATIC, LIQUID FLAVORING AGENTS that require infusing roots, barks, herbs, botanicals, spices, seeds, flowers, and fruit peels in alcohol. Aromatic bitters are added to drinks in dashes, not consumed by themselves; are high in alcohol content; and have very concentrated flavors. As such, they are considered non-potable and are sold with different regulations and taxes than potable bitters that are consumed as stand-alones. These non-potable, aromatic bitters are called cocktail bitters or aromatic cocktail bitters.

Bitters have been used for centuries here and abroad for stomach ailments and respiratory issues, as well as a host of other maladies. The history of alcohol and medicine is full of examples of happy accidents, and the discovery of the healing properties of bitter plants is likely an example of one. Scientists know that animals are drawn to bitter-tasting plants when they are sick, and current thinking is that early humans observed ailing animals eating bitter plants and followed suit.

Bitters have always been an irreplaceable part of the cocktail and are intertwined with its history.

Colonial Americans used to take bitters alone for their medicinal properties, but they were adding bitters to alcohol by the late 1700s. They were big on bitters for breakfast. The very first printed definition of the cocktail (page 55) listed bitters. The explosion of creativity that fueled the Golden Age of the Cocktail ceased abruptly with Prohibition, and bitters suffered greatly for the remainder of the century as a result. In 2003, there were only a handful of commercially available bitters; now, they number in the hundreds, with no signs of slowing down. It is interesting to note that many of the highly bitter botanicals in bitters, such as gentian, have been used medicinally for thousands of years. Some were even listed on ancient Egyptian medical papyri.

Bitters bottle by artist Dorothy Brennan (circa 1939).

## Must-Have Historic Bitters

- **ANGOSTURA AROMATIC BITTERS:** Established in 1824, Angostura has a recognizable yellow cap and oversized paper label (likely a mistake made somewhere along the way and never changed). Angostura doesn't actually contain angostura tree bark, although other bitters do. But Angostura was lawsuit happy, and successful, maintaining exclusive rights to the name, which came from the Venezuelan town where German doctor Johann Gottlieb Benjamin Siegert created it. Early on, sailors took Siegert's bitters for seasickness. Angostura's secret original formula is guarded by only five people.

- **PEYCHAUD'S BITTERS:** Created by New Orleans apothecary Antoine Amedie Peychaud, some consider Peychaud's to be the first commercial bitters. Peychaud was a Creole immigrant from Haiti. He used an old family recipe to devise his bitters and began dispensing it at his New Orleans apothecary starting in 1838. The city's most famous cocktail, the Sazerac, called for Peychaud's, and people began requesting the bitters by name. Along with Angostura, it is one of the few bitters brands that survived Prohibition.

If your drink just doesn't quite sparkle, it is probably missing bitters. We love our bitters, and we developed our own line of proprietary bitters with exotic healing ingredients from around the world.

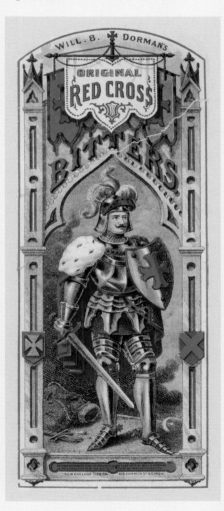

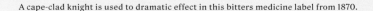

A cape-clad knight is used to dramatic effect in this bitters medicine label from 1870.

# APOTHEKE: ROOTED IN PLANT-BASED MEDICINE

**S**INCE THE DAWN OF HUMAN CIVILIZATION, PLANTS HAVE healed and cured us.

Plants caught the attention of several ancient cultures, including the Aztecs, and were in the medicinal manuals of the Chinese as well as medieval herbals. Herbals are books that describe the medicinal and other properties of plants, often accompanied with illustrations. Some botanists and explorers went on bioprospecting journeys to bring back exotic plants from foreign lands, in hopes of discovering new medicines, and medieval societies took their pharmacopeia endeavors seriously. Some early herbals went on to shape medical views for thousands of years. Many of them went through various translations, from Arabic to Latin and eventually to English, a testament to their profound and lasting influence.

Traditional Chinese medicine, with its long and rich relationship with plants, has been practiced for at least 2,500 years. Verbal and written stories can be traced back even further, to 4,000 years ago, with herbal collection and exploration that helped form the basis of later *materia medica*.

The ancient Indian Vedas—texts that transmit knowledge from generation to generation, including that of Ayurvedic medicine and its use of healing plants— have origins from around 4500 to 2500 BCE. The Atharva Veda praises medicinal plants, but scientists long doubted the text's use as a history of the practice of medicine: it mentions leprosy, and there was no evidence that leprosy existed at that time. In 2009, however, the discovery of a skeleton from 4,000 years ago proved the existence of the disease at that time. This discovery gave new meaning and legitimacy to the record of plants and medicine in ancient India.

*The fever that comes on every third day, that intermits on every third day, that comes continually and that comes in Autumn, fever that is cold and hot and that comes in Summer—destroy him, oh Plant!*

—HYMN TO PLANTS IN THE ATHARVA VEDA

The ancient Babylonians and then Egyptians explored a great number of herbs and documented their medicinal applications on clay tablets and papyrus, respectively. We also know a great deal about the widespread use of plants in Greek and Roman cultures during the height of their intellectual development and influence. The works of Hippocrates, Dioscorides, Galen, and others provided the basis for the development of medicine over the subsequent centuries, and they all relied heavily on natural substances as medicines.

One academic study undertook a rather inspired analysis: the author pored over twelve Arabic and European pharmaceutical works spanning over two millennia—from the fifth century BCE to the nineteenth century CE—in order to determine the foundations of medicine. Five main works (written by Galen, Hippocrates, Dioscorides, Aulus Cornelius Celsus, and Paul of Aegina) formed the pillars of Western pharmaceutical thought for two thousand years, so the author set out to find patterns in their simples (medicinal materials). There were 405 simples identified in the five sources, and 78 percent of these were plants. Of the thirty-one simples they had in common, twenty-six were plants. These included cinnamon, pepper, figs, rose, and cassia. Four of the five manuscripts cited wine as a preservative, solvent, and medicine.

As expected, the plants often came from the Mediterranean world, but they also came from Africa and East Asia. This highlighted the far-reaching impacts of the spice trade and trade routes among the regions, which included the Silk Roads, the Cinnamon Route, and the Incense Roads.

## FROM THE ANCIENTS TO NOW:
## MEDICINAL PLANTS ACROSS TIME

We may laugh or cringe at many of the primitive practices of early medical interventions, such as the use of viper skins, animal organs, lead, and bloodletting. But we must give credit where credit is due: even though they had no means of deciphering how or why the plants worked, ancient medical practitioners and apothecaries got it right in a lot of cases. In fact, many of the plants that debuted in *materia medica* thousands of years ago are still used medicinally today. The following botanicals were used in ancient Sumerian, Egyptian, Greek, Roman, Chinese, and/or Indian medicine, and are still widely used in modern medicine:

ALMOND • ALOE • BEETS • CARAWAY • CARDAMOM • CASSIA
CELERY • CHAMOMILE • CINNAMON • CORIANDER • FENNEL
FIGS • GENTIAN • GINGER • HONEY • HYSSOP • JUNIPER
LICORICE • MARJORAM • ORRIS ROOT • PEPPER • PEPPERMINT
POMEGRANATE • RHUBARB • ROSE • ROSEMARY • SAFFRON
SENNA • TURMERIC • WORMWOOD

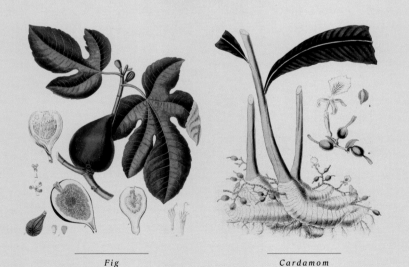

*Fig*                              *Cardamom*

# RISE OF THE APOTHECARY

**T**HE TERM *APOTHECARY* IS DERIVED FROM THE LATIN WORD *apotheca* ("storehouse") and the Greek word *apothēkē*. *Apothecary* originally referred to an individual who prepared compounds, filled prescriptions, and sold medicines. It evolved to also refer to the stores that sold herbs, spices, and wines—essentially the equivalent of a pharmacy or drugstore.

Before there were pharmacists doling out mass-produced synthetic prescriptions in drugstores, apothecaries-cum-wizards crafted custom-made botanical tinctures, tonics, cordials, elixirs, and potions. They used alcohol to preserve the plant components and draw out their healing properties.

Apothecaries inhabited diverse and valued roles in their communities; they were at once pharmacists, chemists, herbalists, surgeons, medical practitioners, caregivers, and midwives. As such, apothecaries needed to have a deep knowledge of healing plants and how to compound ingredients to make the best remedy for a patient's

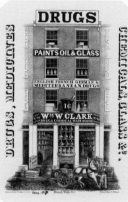

specific malady. Apothecaries served both patients and physicians.

The first apothecary shops appeared as far back as 754 in Baghdad, where apothecaries sold wines, syrups, perfumes, herbs, and spices alongside medicines in street markets. By the eleventh century, apothecaries could be found in Islamic Spain. During the fifteenth and sixteenth centuries, apothecaries solidified their valued status in the community, and they remained popular until the late nineteenth century.

Apothecary shops had very unusual methods for distinguishing themselves to passersby. In addition to the standard

William Clark's druggist shop, at 16 North Fifth Street in Philadelphia.

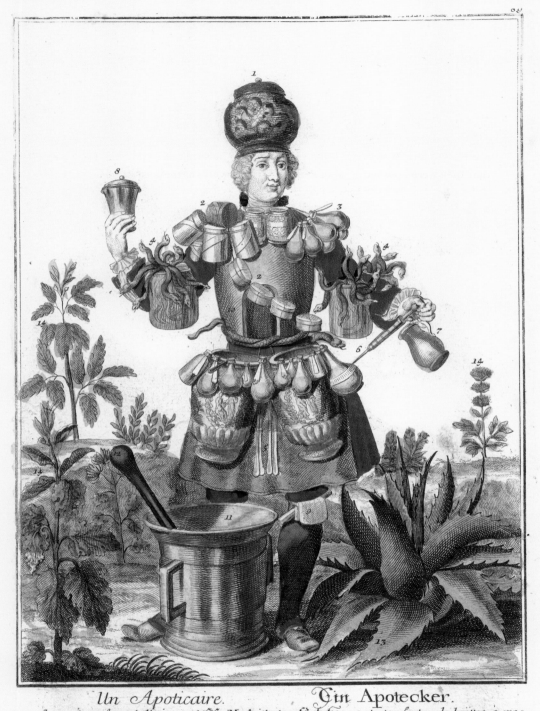

## Un Apoticaire.   Ein Apotecker.

1. vase pour la conserve de l'opiat. 1. Gefäße Medrithat aufzuheben. 2. toutes sortes de boettes à me-
decines. 2. schachtelen und Büchsen mit Arzeneyen. 3. verres à medecine. 3. Glaßlen mit Arzeneyen.
4. lesars, viperes, serpens. 4. Schlangen oder Ottern, vipern. 5. patule. 5. Spatllen. 6. ciringue. 6. Sprützen.
7. cruche. 7. ein Krügle. 8. goblet d'or à prendre medecine. 8. ein goldenes Becherl zum einnehmen. 9.
recepte. 9. recepte. 10. fourneau. 10. ein Ofen. 11. mortier. 11. ein Mörser. 12. pilon. 12. der Stößel.
13. aloe. 13. aloe. 14. Simples. 14. allerley zur Arzeney dienliche Kräuter.

Cum Priv. Maj                                                    Mart. Engelbrecht. excud. A. V.

shelves of bottled elixirs and medicine jars, apothecaries would often decorate their shops with exotica, like taxidermic alligators. Many apothecaries placed show globes, also called carboys, in their front windows to attract customers and signal that they were apothecary shops. Show globes were decorative and appealing, filled with red, green, and blue liquids and illuminated from behind. Records show that they were common in the nineteenth and twentieth centuries, but their history may reach even further back. The absence of a clear origin story has invited several myths.

> *Apothecary apprenticeships included learning about fermentation and distillation techniques and a vast array of herbs. Not surprisingly, apothecaries were mostly men. But legal records show at least three women rose to prominence in the apothecary world after their husbands died and they were legally recognized as apothecary shop owners.*

Apothecaries firmly took hold in England in the fourteenth century. Although they were well established earlier, the first recorded mention of an apothecary in England was in 1345 in Thomas Rymer's *Foedera*, wherein it states that Coursus de Gangeland attended to a sick King Edward III and is called "an Apothecary of London." The Worshipful Society of Apothecaries of London was incorporated by royal charter in 1617 as a City Livery Company and remains active today. It founded the

Chelsea Physic Garden in 1673, and has granted medical licenses since 1815. British mystery writer Agatha Christie passed the Society of Apothercaries' Assistants' Examination in 1917.

The society's coat of arms includes a rhinoceros as the crest (the powdered horn of the rhinoceros was thought to be medicinal). The motto on the coat of arms, quoted from Ovid's *Metamorphoses*, succinctly encapsulates apothecaries' philosophy: "I am spoken of all over the world as one who brings help." This certainly proved to be true during the Great Plague in 1665. When most of London's physicians died or fled, apothecaries stayed to tend to the sick.

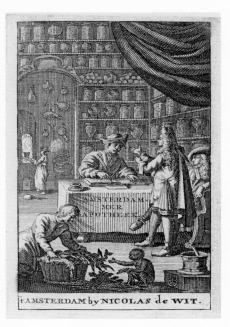

tAMSTERDAM by NICOLAS de WIT.

---

OPPOSITE: An apothecary with the costume and tools of his craft—note the aloe plant and the vipers—was part of a series of eighteenth-century illustrations by Martin Engelbrecht. • ABOVE: Apothecaries of yore wove a tapestry of cures, draped in mystery and drenched in flair. This is a typical apothecary shop in Amsterdam.

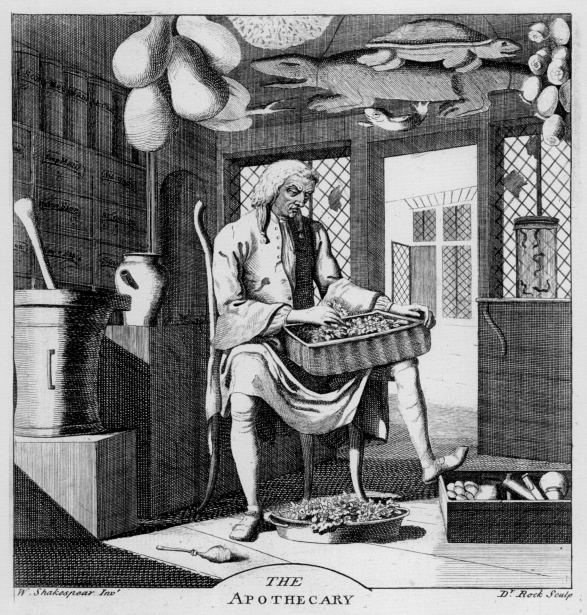

## THE
## APOTHECARY

W. Shakespear Inv.

D.' Rock Sculp.

I do remember an Apothecary,
And hereabouts he dwells, which late I noted
In tatter'd Weeds, with overwhelming Brows,
Culling of Simples; meager were his Looks,
Sharp Misery had worn him to the Bones:
And in his needy Shop a Tortoise hung,

An Alligator stuft, and other Skins
Of ill shap'd Fishes, and about his Shelves
A beggarly Account of empty Boxes;
Green earthen Pots, Bladders, and musty Seeds,
Remnants of Packthread, and old Cakes of Roses
Where thinly scattered to make up a shew.

Accord.ᵈ to y.ᵉ Act. To be had of T. Ewart facing Old Slaughters Coffee House S.ᵗ Martins Lane Long Acre.        Price

# TO WHOM OR WHAT CAN WE THANK FOR THE COCKTAIL?

**T**HE NEXT TIME YOU TAKE A SIP OF A COCKTAIL, THINK of this: you are drinking the result of millions of years of plant evolution and tapping into the rich botanical and chemical knowledge base of societies around the world. Fabled medieval alchemists gave us the apparatus that made spirits possible, and some of the most famous early thought leaders recorded prescriptions for plants and alcohol on clay tablets and in hand-drawn manuscripts that transcended time and culture. Medicinal cocktails connect us to ancient healing wisdom.

Colonial America popularized adding bitters to alcohol, as well as the cocktail. There is speculation that the cocktail was technically being consumed in London by 1750, in the form of punches served individually, but the renegade Americans certainly took the concept and ran with it.

In Europe, the word *cocktail* first appeared in London's *Morning Post and Gazetteer* in 1798. On the other side of the Atlantic, the first printed mention of a cocktail was in 1803 in a New Hampshire newspaper titled the *Farmer's Cabinet*: "Drank a glass of cocktail—excellent for the head. . . . Call'd at the Doct's. found Burnham—he looked very wise—drank another glass of cocktail."

Cocktails owe their very existence to the history of alcohol as medicine, since the first written recipe included bitters: in 1806, a Hudson, New York, newspaper, *The Balance and Columbian Repository*, listed spirits, bitters, sugar, and water as ingredients of the cocktail. Some speculate that the name *cocktail* is related to its start as a morning drink, the rooster (cock) being annoying in the morning. Other stories are ridiculous, such as the claim that Antoine Peychaud (the New Orleans apothecary who created Peychaud's Bitters) invented the cocktail. He was three years old in 1806.

---

The lettering in this 1750 engraving is from Romeo's monologue in William Shakespeare's *Romeo and Juliet*, where he reflects on getting an elixir of death from an apothecary.

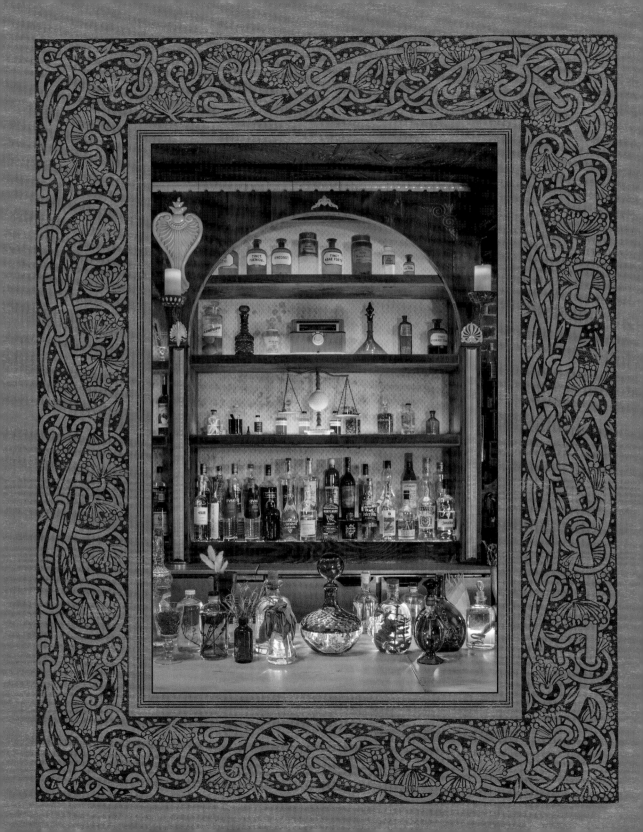

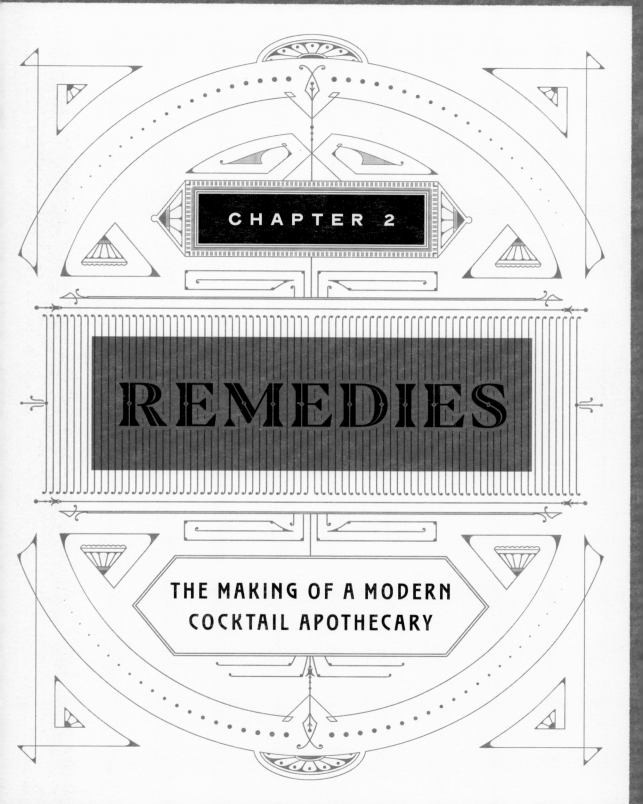

# CHAPTER 2

# REMEDIES

## THE MAKING OF A MODERN COCKTAIL APOTHECARY

**E**VERY COCKTAIL NEEDS A STARTING POINT, AND THERE are six main base spirits that form the foundation upon which cocktails are built: brandy (Cognac and pisco), gin, tequila and mezcal, rum, vodka, and whiskey (bourbon, Scotch, rye, moonshine). You'll also need modifying alcohols, which are generally lower proof spirits and liqueurs that complement the base spirit by adding flavor and body. We like to use vermouth, Aperol, amaro, Bénédictine, rosolio, sake, baijiu, and aquavit. We also enjoy finishing cocktails with toppers of Champagne (a short pour of bubbles to fill and add fizz) and floats (a delicate pour of red wine over the back side of a bar spoon that adds colorful layering). We like to get creative with absinthe and have found special ways to work its medicinal magic into our offerings.

### PROOF AND ABV

**D**uring the sixteenth century, the British navy provided its sailors with beer on long voyages as it kept longer than water—and kept morale up. But as even beer would spoil during lengthy trips, they switched to rum. Later, the powers that be devised a sneaky way of getting scurvy-fighting citrus into sailors, while avoiding the neglect of duties that frequently occurred when sailors were handed pure pints of rum: they created a grog with rum, water, lime juice, and sugar.

In the eighteenth century, suspicious sailors began insisting on testing their rum rations for proof that they weren't watered down. They would mix rum into gunpowder and try to ignite it. If the mixture didn't catch on fire, it didn't have enough alcohol content; it was underproof. Someone later discovered that rum only needed to be 57 percent alcohol by volume (ABV) in order to ignite, a ratio of approximately 7:4. In the United States, this was rounded to the much easier formula of 2:1, so that a 100-proof bottle of rum is 50 percent ABV. The United Kingdom retained the original standard, and a 100-proof bottle has 57 percent alcohol.

*Proof is only a rough measure of alcohol content, and legally, a liquor label must list its ABV, which is the alcohol content as a percentage of volume.*

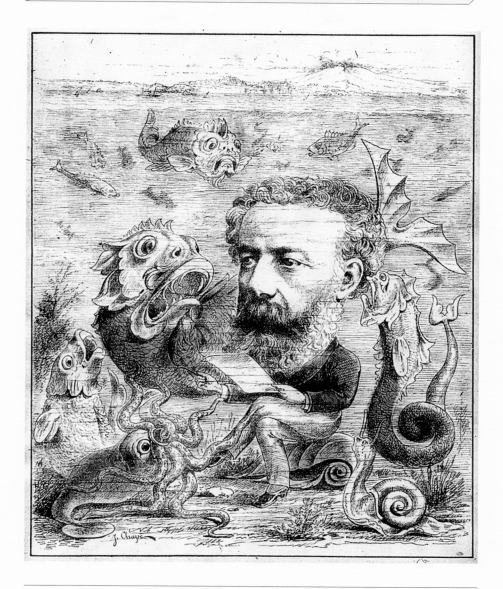

PREVIOUS SPREAD: Behind our glowing marble bar in New York is a hand-carved archway displaying antique bottles. • ABOVE: Ancient explorers took to the seas on epic bioprospecting voyages, braving the ocean's majestic but turbulent powers to find exotic medicinal plants. The deep sea is also where we get ABV.

# BASE SPIRITS

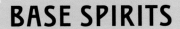

BRANDY

NOTES FROM NICOLAS O'CONNOR

*I find brandy to be one of the more challenging spirits to master. The wide array of varietals reflects the entire spectrum of the palate, which creates plenty of optionality. Whether brandy is the featured ingredient or a complement, it provides a unique, full-proof option for cocktail creation. While experimenting, I often turn to different types of brandy in an effort to discover the proper depth and flavor notes that I'm searching for. Its versatility—the floral nature of pisco, the crisp sweetness of applejack, or the woody notes of Cognac—means it can be mixed with any number of fresh elements. It also works incredibly well in blends with other full-proof spirits, adding new flavor twists to the base spirit.*

Brandy can be thought of as a distilled wine. It can be distilled from any fermented fruit, including apples, cherries, peaches, pears, and plums, but most commonly wine grapes. Some brandies are well known for the deep flavors they develop from aging in wooden casks, though not all types of brandies are aged.

## PLANTS AND PROOF

*Plants:* Any fruit, usually wine grapes
*Proof:* 60–120 (30–60% ABV)

## MEDICINAL PROPERTIES

One of the reasons brandy and other spirits are viewed as curatives is that early medicinal models drew upon the philosophy of Aristotle (and later, Hippocrates) that human health was composed of four dimensions: cold, heat, dry, and moist. People thought that the heat associated with spirits—aqua vitae was even referred to as *aqua ardens*, or "burning water," due to the heat required to distill it—was appropriate for maladies in the cold realm. Brandy was recommended for elderly persons' cooling bodies, but not for already-warm youngsters. Later on, however, brandy and other spirits became widely prescribed for fevers, pneumonia, and other ailments. Some physicians even recommended giving babies a bit of brandy.

Of all the base spirits, brandy is most closely linked to medicine. Early distillations of wine were undertaken in order to create medicinal tonics. Physicians and apothecaries used it as a stand-alone healing agent and as a vehicle for other medicinal substances. Belief in brandy's restorative effects, for both specific maladies and as a general tonic, was virtually ubiquitous until the nineteenth century.

Physicians and apothecaries trumpeted brandy's health-granting effects.

Brandy was deployed for heart disease, gout, headaches, deafness, and countless other physical ailments. It was touted as a remedy not only for sicknesses, but also for concerns about appearances and emotional health.

The spirit was believed to arrest aging and prolong youth. People who could afford it started taking it every morning for its energizing and warming effects, and some Europeans still do.

Thanks to the polyphenols in the wood barrels they're aged in, brandies have high levels of antioxidant activity. Analyses of brandy's disease-fighting effects have shown that its polyphenolic makeup is altered from being stored in polyphenol-rich wood.

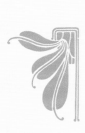
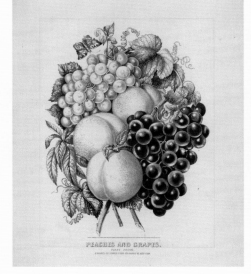

PEACHES AND GRAPES.

# GIN

### NOTES FROM NICOLAS O'CONNOR

*Gin is great to use in cocktails that feature big, bold flavors. Gin provides a nice botanical accompaniment to strong sour, sweet, and savory ingredients that tend to drown out other flavors and dominate the palate. I particularly love how gin can elevate fresh ingredients by softening their impact and rounding the combined flavor of the entire cocktail while maintaining its own character. The wide range of gins available today provide a variety of impressions to work with, like floral, botanical, and even spicy. Gin also makes big flavors from fruits, vegetables, and citrus stand out. The taste of gin is a complex denouement on the back of the palate, which allows gin's essence to linger. I like to combine gin with bright flavors that are easily identified, like common fruits and vegetables, but aren't generally associated with cocktails. I appreciate gin's ability to elevate recognizable flavors while creating a unique cocktail.*

Gin is a neutral spirit, often grain-based, unaged, and high proof. To be technically considered gin, it must be flavored mainly with juniper. Grains tend to provide the best base for this spirit, but gin can be distilled from anything that has enough fermentable carbohydrates. It is often a mix of barley, rye, and corn or wheat. Gin is rectified (distilled twice or more) to produce the base spirit and then flavored with juniper berries and other botanicals. Some gins use up to a dozen botanicals for flavoring, and more than one hundred different botanicals have been used in different combinations.

Gin is characterized by its numerous botanical ingredients, which can include almond, angelica root, anise, bay leaf, cardamom, cassia, cinnamon, citrus peel (such as sweet orange peel or lemon peel), cocoa nibs, coriander, cubeb, fennel, ginger, grains of paradise, lavender, licorice, nutmeg, orris root, and rose. After juniper berries, coriander is the second-most critical flavoring in the majority of gins. Coriander is one of the most ancient remedies in history, with Egyptian hieroglyphs documenting its use in medicine. Angelica root is the third-most prevalent botanical used in gin, and it has a dry, earthy flavor.

## PLANTS AND PROOF

*Plants:* Barley, rye, wheat, corn, juniper, and an assortment of botanicals
*Proof:* 80–114 (40–57% ABV)

## MEDICINAL PROPERTIES

Gin was originally created as a medicine, possibly to cure stomach ailments. The spirit was also thought to be effective in fighting diseases, such as scurvy and malaria.

The classic gimlet cocktail has its origins in gin's link to medicine. The British Parliament mandated in 1867 that certain ships provide lemon or lime juice to sailors as a way of providing scurvy-fighting vitamin C. Sir Thomas Desmond Gimlette, the Royal Navy's doctor, devised the idea of combining Navy Strength (57% ABV) gin and Rose's Lime Juice Cordial to "fortify" and "immunize," respectively. Thus, the gimlet was born. We have our own take on the gimlet (page 191).

In the 1800s, companies figured out how to make quinine—a bitter-tasting, malaria-fighting compound from Peruvian cinchona bark—easy to ingest: tonic water. Tonic is carbonated water with quinine. By the end of the century, British colonists had discovered the compatibility of tonic and gin, and the rest is history. So you could say that gin technically helped fight a major disease.

Juniper, a member of the ancient cypress family, is one of the oldest medicines still in use today. It is a stimulant, weight-loss aid, and pain reliever. It's also known for its diuretic effects.

In the second century CE, Greek physician Galen linked juniper berries to liver and kidney cleansing. In the thirteenth century, Belgian theologian Thomas van Cantimpré suggested boiling juniper berries in wine or rainwater to help with stomach pain.

In a 1652 publication, Nicholas Culpeper, an English apothecary and man of the common people, recommended juniper berry for several illnesses, such as gout, and for improving memory and sight. Always a rebel, he published his recommendations in a medical guide specifically created to help people who could not pay for apothecary services or read Latin, which was still the standard language for medical works and restricted most medical information to physicians and the upper echelon.

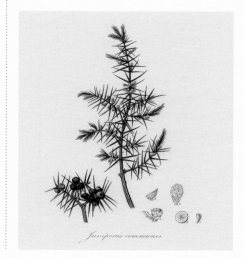

*Juniperus communis.*

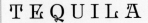

# TEQUILA

## NOTES FROM NICOLAS O'CONNOR

*When working with tequila, I keep its rich golden flavor in my frontal lobes. I appreciate how it maintains its footing, even when equally balanced with other hearty ingredients. I find it mixes effortlessly with sour, sweet, salty, and spicy flavors. It elevates flavors while providing its own distinct aftertaste. Crafting cocktails with delicate herbs and spices can be challenging, but incorporating strong fruits or vegetables that pair nicely with tequila makes it less difficult. This provides a solid base that allows the delicate flavors to easily accent the cocktail.*

The Mexican spirit tequila is distinguished from mezcal in several ways: It must be made entirely from a particular cultivar of *Agave tequilana*—the "Weber Blue"—in a designated area around the state of Jalisco. The hand-harvesting that characterizes mezcal is replaced by large-field farming, and the underground roasting is replaced by heating and steaming in an oven. When choosing a tequila, make sure to get 100 percent agave tequila (it may also carry the label 100 percent *de agave* or 100 percent *puro de agave*); avoid bottles labeled mixto.

### PLANTS AND PROOF

*Plants:* Agave (*Agave tequilana*—only the "Weber Blue" variety)
*Proof:* 70–110 (35–55% ABV)

### MEDICINAL PROPERTIES

The agave in tequila has many healing qualities. The blue agave's sugar, a fructan, had its chemical structure described for the first time a few years ago, and scientists are looking into its potential for diabetes-related applications.

> *Mexicans believe that tequila can help fight the common cold.*

# MEZCAL

### NOTES FROM NICOLAS O'CONNOR

*Mezcal operates much like tequila. Both spirits work in tandem with the strongest flavors in a cocktail. They uplift while maintaining their own dominant presence. Mezcal distinguishes itself by adding a strong, smoky flavor with earthy hints from the natural terroir of Oaxaca. When I want to create a mezcal-based cocktail, I start by making it with a pliable tequila as the base spirit. The clean body of tequila allows me to more easily understand how the ingredients interact and find balance. Once I am happy with flavor and body, I simply replace the tequila with mezcal. With the knowledge I gain by first making the cocktail with tequila, I know swapping in the mezcal will result in the same flavor, but with more depth on the palate from a beautiful, smoky-savory layer.*

Mezcal is a Mexican spirit made from the roasted heart of the agave plant (piña). Mexican laws state that to be able to put mezcal on the label, the spirit must come from Oaxaca, Guerrero, Durango, San Luis Potosí, or Zacatecas. High-quality mezcals usually indicate the origin village and agave species. Unlike tequila, which is restricted to one particular cultivar of *Agave tequilana* ("Weber Blue"), mezcal can be made from thirty different types of agave, the most common being *espadin*. Oaxaca is home to twenty-three different types of agave. At the heart of any mezcal is its ancient method of production, often passed down from generation to generation, and its small-batch, handcrafted style.

## PLANTS AND PROOF
*Plants:* Agave
*Proof:* 80–100 (40–50% ABV)

## MEDICINAL PROPERTIES
Agave is a natural stimulant. Mexicans have used agave for medicinal purposes for hundreds of years.

Research has shown the fructans of certain types of agave have prebiotic effects, which can be used to prevent gastrointestinal diseases and promote gut health. Agavin sugar from agave is being investigated for its weight-loss and diabetic applications. Some also believe mezcal contains aphrodisiac qualities. Mexican harvesters and producers see mezcal as a spirit with many medicinal benefits.

# RUM

### NOTES FROM NICOLAS O'CONNOR

*Rum is the most regionally specific spirit and has a rich history of tiki culture. When I taste rum, I'm immediately transported to the tropical Caribbean. I often play on this, and my rum creations end up quite exotic. I love how rum functions with sour and bitter flavors. I especially like to take advantage of how the inherent sweet notes from sugarcane provide a natural balance to sour and bitter flavors. By relying on rum's natural sweetness, I eliminate the need for excess sweeteners that cocktails so often require. Rum is slightly denser than gin or vodka, but not as heavy as tequila or whiskey. Thus, I find rum is a great way to introduce richer layers to fresh cocktails without dominating the other ingredients.*

Rum is a spirit distilled from sugarcane or its byproducts (molasses, fresh or evaporated sugarcane juice, sugarcane syrup, crystallized sugars). First created in Barbados in the mid-1600s, it remains a mainly Caribbean-produced, molasses-based spirit. Rum is a spirit for which the six different types have diverse tastes and characters.

Importantly, aging rum in wooden barrels in the tropical climate of the Caribbean changes everything. It is estimated that aging occurs two to three times faster for rum in the Caribbean than for a liquor aging in a colder climate. This makes it possible to produce a more mature, rich spirit in less time—which also drives down costs.

### PLANTS AND PROOF
*Plants:* Sugarcane
*Proof:* 60–151 (30–75.5% ABV)

### MEDICINAL PROPERTIES
Rum has been widely used as a painkiller. During the American Revolutionary War, army officers were given rum and brandy for pain, and soldiers received a daily ration of rum. Colonial Americans used rum for a range of illnesses as well.

In 1970, former Royal Navy sailors went in front of the British parliament to defend the health- and morale-boosting benefits of rum when it looked like daily rum rations would be taken away, but their efforts were unsuccessful.

*The British navy stopped doling out rum rations ("tots") in 1970, but the link between the navy, rum, and proof is reflected in the fact that some rums and other liquors with 57 percent ABV are still sold with the label "Navy Strength."*

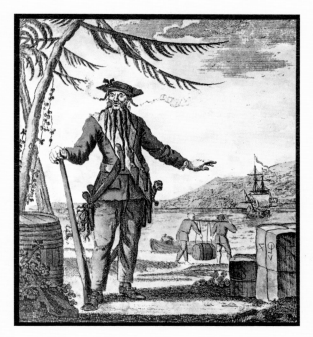

Rum is thought to relax the body and reduce stress. The stress-relieving properties of rum may be the reason for its inclusion in so many tropical, vacation-reminiscent drinks.

Sugarcane, rum's raw material, has medicinal properties that were recognized by the ancients. Babylonian medical tablets provide a recipe for a colic treatment that included sweet reed (which is similar to sugarcane) and other botanicals infused into wine. In Dioscorides's famous *De materia medica*, he noted that sugarcane was helpful for the intestines, stomach, and kidneys. Sugarcane was transported from its native Bengal coast to gardens, where it could be cultivated for its sugar water, followed by sugar. It was seen as a therapeutic agent, appearing in doctors' prescriptions in Sassanid Persia. In the tenth century, the Salerno School included sugar in its pharmacopeia.

Molasses is the most common rum base, and it helps with mineral absorption in the body. This facilitates growth and bone development. Darker molasses, such as blackstrap molasses, is the healthiest type.

Blackbeard the Pirate (aka Captain Teach) in Daniel Defoe's *A General History of the Lives and Adventures of the Most Famous Highwaymen, Murderers, Street-Robbers, &c. to which is added, a genuine account of the voyages and plunders of the most notorious pyrates* (circa 1736).

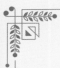
# VODKA

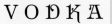

NOTES FROM NICOLAS O'CONNOR

*A widely used and essential spirit for cocktail creation, vodka is often misunderstood. Vodka's lack of its own true flavor provides an empty canvas for many lighter ingredients to shine but still gives the required base strength. When I create a cocktail using an exotic or rare ingredient that I've never worked with before, I always begin with vodka. The neutral base allows more subtle flavors to maintain their character and remain present on the palate. I pair vodka with uncommon flavors because it allows one to focus on exciting new tastes and sensations.*

Vodka is a clear, neutral, odorless spirit that can be made from a mash of myriad botanicals, including rye, wheat, corn, barley, potatoes, quinoa, and soybeans. It can be made from anything with enough carbohydrates to allow fermentation; ingredients can even include those traditionally associated with other spirits, such as sugarcane, sugar beets, grapes, honey, apples, tree sap, and milk. It contains very few congeners, and it is unaged.

## PLANTS AND PROOF

*Plants:* Rye, wheat, potatoes, corn, barley, sugarcane, grapes, honey, apples, and tree sap

*Proof:* 75–176 (37.5–88% ABV)

## MEDICINAL PROPERTIES

Vodka has been linked to medicinal uses since its inception. Russians would infuse their vodka with herbs, berries, fruit, spices, and honey to help with the taste but also to boost the medicinal value. Russians use vodka with peppers for a cold and with salt for stomach issues.

Vodka is an antiseptic, can increase blood flow and circulation, and can lower blood sugar levels. It has sedative and anesthetizing qualities as well.

The native Anishinaabe people say that vodka can help relax the throat and is a useful addition to homemade rose tonics and cough syrup, which also help prevent colds.

> *Congeners are a side effect of fermentation caused by the random couplings of molecules and yeast enzymes: they can include esters, terpenes, and volatile phenolics, as well as undesirable substances.*

# WHISKEY

NOTES FROM NICOLAS O'CONNOR

*Whiskeys, more than any other spirit category, maintain their strength and character when mixed with other ingredients. That is why they are so frequently featured in Apotheke's stirred, spirit-forward cocktails. The rich complexity of whiskeys carries the base of the cocktail while complementary ingredients balance and build on the whiskey's unique flavor. When working whiskeys into plant-based, shaken cocktails, where it shares the stage with other ingredients, it's important to use vivid, bold botanicals. Prominent sweet and sour notes that hit the palate early blend well with robust whiskeys. I love mixing whiskey with bright berries, larger flavorful fruits, and tart citrus that hold court to the strength of the whiskey. Subtle notes and flavors can get lost, feel separated, and be difficult to balance.*

Whiskey is basically distilled beer, minus the hops, aged in oak barrels. It can be made from whatever grain makes the most sense to the distiller, based on the grains native to the area: corn, rye, wheat, or malted barley.

Whiskey (also known as whisky in some countries) is basically an umbrella term that encompasses Scotch, bourbon, rye, and other whiskey. Scotch is whisky from Scotland, with a distinct style and production process from Irish whiskey. Bourbon is an American whiskey made from corn. And rye is a rye-based whiskey, often from the United States but not exclusively so.

Like Europe's other traditional spirits, such as aquavit, brandy, gin, and vodka, whiskey dates to the late Middle Ages and Renaissance. And like other spirits, the exact date and location of its birth remain hotly contested.

## PLANTS AND PROOF
*Plants:* Barley, corn, rye, wheat
*Proof:* 70–140 (35–70% ABV)

## MEDICINAL PROPERTIES
Whiskey has been used as an anesthetic since its beginnings. Some of whiskey's medicinal qualities may be due to the phenolic compounds in the oak barrels it is aged in. Whiskey is high in ellagic acid, an antioxidant with cancer-fighting potential.

The U.S. Pharmacopeia listed whiskey as an official drug until 1917. Further investigation reveals that it was voted to be removed in 1915, not because of questions of its appropriateness as a medicine, but because of concerns that the governing body could not accurately give standards for a product that was sometimes adulterated.

During Prohibition, whiskey and other liquors were granted exemption under the Volstead Act if prescribed as medicines. Some whiskey distilleries were able to stay open to meet this demand, but others

shuttered and struggled to rebound after the law was repealed. In 1921, researchers and advocates conducted a large-scale survey of American doctors to assess their attitudes toward medicinal alcohol. They were asked about whiskey and beer as therapeutics. The results were intended to convince lawmakers and add to the policy debate. Fifty-one percent of doctors considered whiskey to be a therapeutic agent, and 25 percent felt this way about beer.

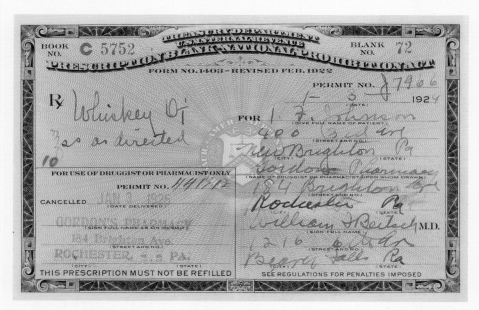

After being granted permits to dispense liquor, doctors prescribed eight million gallons of medicinal alcohol in Prohibition's first year.

# GOGGINS HOUR

**W**E HAD THE PRIVILEGE OF PARTNERING WITH THE inimitable Walton Goggins and Mulholland Distilling at Apotheke LA in February 2018.

The amazing and magnetic actor Walton Goggins is a fan of Apotheke and a partner at Mulholland Distilling. He collaborated with Nicolas O'Connor, Apotheke mixology director, to create three specialty cocktails for an exciting evening event that was coined Goggins Hour.

One of these formulas can be found in Part II (Sunburned Hand of the Man, page 155), and we're including an exclusive recipe on the next page.

Mulholland Distilling was born in 2016. Goggins and founder/partner Matthew Alper set out to capture the unique essence of LA and bring artisanal spirits to LA and beyond, channeling *The Spirit of Los Angeles*™. Their spirits have won a plethora of awards, and their focus on quality and craft is evident in the fact that they have dedicated years to developing the best possible flavor profiles.

Mulholland offers the following artisanal spirits—all blended and bottled just outside of downtown LA:

- **AMERICAN WHISKEY**
  Award-winning, 100 proof, with maple and sweet corn flavors.
- **NEW WORLD GIN**
  Double Gold Medal, with undertones of cucumber, lavender, and lime.
- **MULHOLLAND VODKA**
  Gluten-free, 100 percent non-GMO corn.

The craft spirits company has had numerous features in major publications like the *Daily Beast*, *Eater LA*, *Fast Company*, *Hollywood Reporter*, *Playboy*, and *Variety*.

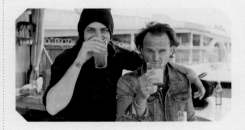

*For more information, see:*
WWW.MULHOLLANDDISTILLING.COM

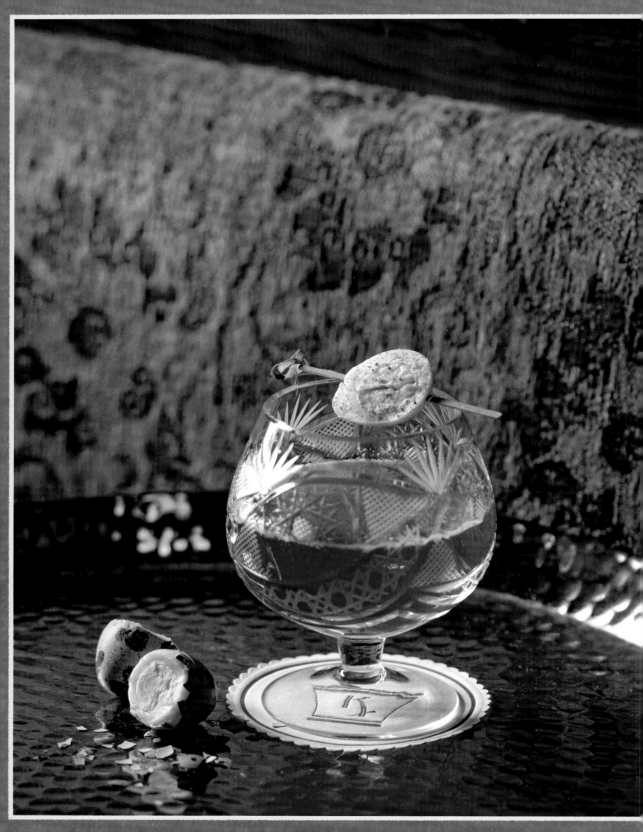

# NUMBER THREE
# HOLD THE HASH BROWNS

CREATED BY WALTON GOGGINS AND NICOLAS O'CONNOR

*Inspired by Walton's favorite Waffle House order, Number Three Hold the Hash Browns is a savory ode to classic Americana. A simple yet bold profile, it takes stirred cocktails in a new direction while presenting familiar flavors.*

## FORMULA

1 hard-boiled quail egg

2 ounces Mulholland American Whiskey

1 bar spoon horseradish

¼ bar spoon agave nectar

Pinch Old Bay Seasoning

## TOOLS

Jigger

Mixing glass

Bar spoon

Hawthorne strainer

Rocks glass

## EXECUTION

Hard-boil a quail egg. Pour the whiskey into a mixing glass and add the horseradish and agave nectar. Stir until the horseradish is dissolved. Strain into a rocks glass over fresh ice. Peel the egg and cut it in half, sprinkle it with Old Bay Seasoning, skewer it with a toothpick, and place it on the rim of the glass.

# BEHIND THE BAR

**A**NY CREATIVE SPIRIT NEEDS A PLACE TO EXPLORE WHAT it is that drives them. Having the proper tools and environment allows the creative to flourish. Just as an artist needs the right paintbrush, mixology is at its best when you've gotten the details right. With that in mind, we'd like to share the setup we have found successful.

## Tools

### JIGGERS

Jiggers are a mixologist's most important tool. Keeping precise measurements is essential to creating and continually executing well-balanced cocktails. When using finite materials, even a single drop can alter the taste profile. Jiggers can be found in a myriad of shapes and sizes. We use three sizes: 2 fluid ounces/1 fluid ounce, 1½ fluid ounces/¾ fluid ounce, and 1 fluid ounce/½ fluid ounce. This allows us to accurately measure all liquid ingredients to ensure continuity from cocktail to cocktail.

### SHAKER SET / MIXING GLASS and BAR SPOON

When preparing cold cocktails, there are two basic techniques: shaken and stirred.

When shaking a cocktail, the agitation and breakdown of ice adds oxygen and expands the fresh ingredients' molecules, allowing all components to synergize. This method is employed when trying to activate a group of ingredients and creates a balanced, brighter line of flavor. When stirring a cocktail, the lack of expanded molecules and dilution allows for specific ingredients to stand out. Stirring is generally used to highlight full-proof spirits, as each ingredient keeps more of its own identity.

We have our mixologists use the tools that they feel most comfortable with to execute complicated, well-balanced cocktails at a high volume. With shakers, there are two schools of thought, both with pros: in New York, they use a Boston shaker, while in Los Angeles, they use what's called tin on tin. Both are similar in shape and design. The more classic

Boston shaker consists of two parts: a 28-ounce metal cup and a 16-ounce pint glass. The pint glass lets the bartender visually monitor the ingredients during preparation and allows for alteration if any component is off. This is helpful when making large quantities of the same cocktail, as the visual consistency should always remain the same. Tin on tin, or cheater tin, replaces the pint glass with an 18-ounce tin. Shaking with an all-metal construction allows for greater and more consistent cooling than glass. Metal is more flexible than glass, giving it a better grip, as well as a better seal.

Mixing glasses and bar spoons come in a number of varieties. Mixing glasses' shape and size can vary as long as there is ample space to contain all ingredients and a generous amount of ice. The function is to lower the temperature of a mixture without the violent movement of shaking. A bar spoon allows for the ice and liquid to move together, limiting the breakdown of the ice and dilution of the cocktail.

### STRAINERS

We employ three types of strainers: the Hawthorne (with springs), julep (without springs), and tea strainer (for double straining). Each is used to control the mouthfeel of the cocktails by controlling the density and texture of the liquids. The Hawthorne strainer consists of a flat disc to which a coiled spring is affixed. The spring traps large chunks or slivers of ice and other solid ingredients. With a Hawthorne strainer, you can do a light strain.

### MUDDLER

A muddler is used to activate the essences of natural ingredients. They come in many shapes and sizes, all with the purpose of breaking apart the flavor and nutritional characteristics of fresh botanicals. In the case of herbs, it only takes a gentle press to release the essential oils. For fruits, vegetables, and roots, you need to go with a firm push to extract the juices within.

### CITRUS PEELER

While many peels can be done with a knife, the Y-peeler provides an even and uniform cut for your zests and garnishes. It features a sharp, stainless steel blade that glides through tough fruit and vegetable skins. If you're wondering whether a Y-peeler is superior to a traditional straight-blade peeler, the answer is a resounding yes.

### ATOMIZER

An atomizer is a device that produces a fine spray from a liquid. Whether coating a glass or misting the top of a cocktail, an atomizer is a great way to activate and interact with different areas of the palate. Presenting a thought-out smell or "nose" is an essential component to a rounded cocktail.

### DROPPER

Droppers allow for precise distribution of liquids in amounts ranging from ¼ ounce to a single drop. This is useful when using concentrated liquids that greatly modify taste and call for only the smallest amount. Droppers are also used for aesthetic applications due to their ability to control the placement of liquids, such as liquids of different densities, or to draw on top of foams.

## Glassware

We follow the philosophy that all aspects of a cocktail need to be addressed and enhanced to create an all-around experience—it's a thread that seamlessly connects all elements and attacks every sense. From visual to taste, touch to smell, it all makes a difference. An integral piece of this storytelling is the glassware. Different vessels not only attract the eye, but also allow the elevation of the contents within to their utmost potential. In addition to the following glassware, we also use wine, flute, and snifter glasses for our creations. Each was chosen for its elegance; each is used for its function.

### ROCKS GLASS

Rocks glasses, or old-fashioned glasses, are used when presenting a cocktail on ice. Their versatility lends well to both stirred, spirit-forward cocktails and to shaken drinks with fresh ingredients. The key is the slow dilution the ice provides. It sparks the gradual evolution of a cocktail's flavor and maintains a lower temperature throughout consumption.

### COLLINS GLASS

Collins glasses are used for drinks on ice that contain larger proportions of non-alcoholic and bubbly ingredients. The longer and taller design maximizes the carbonated ingredients' effervescence. It's the cocktail version of the flute glass.

### COUPE GLASS

Cocktails without ice belong in an elegant coupe glass. Designated for cocktails that have been thoroughly shaken or chilled and for which any added dilution from ice would flatten flavor and taste. Coupe glasses aren't just pretty for pretty's sake; their large mouth allows the drinker's nose to get close to the surface of the drink and fully enjoy its aromas. This primes the palate even before the liquid hits the taste buds. The long stem prevents the heat from the consumer's hands from affecting the temperature of the drink.

*Cocktails are predominantly water, with one-quarter of this coming from melted ice.*

## Ice

We need ice for two key jobs in making cocktails: diluting and chilling. These seemingly obvious functions of ice are deceptive in their simplicity—they're far more nuanced and physics-driven than the casual observer may think. In developing our ice program, we pay attention to the quality and clarity of the ice, as well as the size. Bigger is generally better when it comes to shaken cocktails; the surface area of small ice cubes can lead to over-dilution, as can be the case with julep or peanut package ice.

Although it's en vogue in the craft cocktail world to work with larger ice forms made from molds, we have found that medium-sized square cubes are best for all-around use. We use Kold Draft machines to make our 1¼-inch cubes in large quantities. The machine has a special design to create clear ice and eliminate the taste that most retail ice molds leave behind. It produces ice of the right size and quality—the ice cubes melt slowly, and they don't break up easily when in a shaker. An added bonus is that these cubes fit in a wide variety of glassware. Ice can also act as a muddler when delicate herbs or berries are part of your recipe.

It sounds counterintuitive, but you don't want your ice to be too cold. It should be close to freezing, but not drastically colder. When you take ice from the freezer, it should look wet and transparent. If it looks dry and opaque, let it sit to warm up to just below freezing. Always remember to shake the water off of your ice before using it. Bypassing this step can lead to a watered-down drink and excess cocktail liquid sticking to the ice.

> *Iced cocktails became possible even before mechanical refrigeration. In the mid-nineteenth century, ice dealers began shipping ice from frozen rivers and lakes—this was clear ice. The ice was able to survive the hot journeys because large volumes of ice melt slower than small volumes.*

## CLEAR ICE vs. CLOUDY ICE

The ice from your freezer is cloudy. This is due to the short amount of time it takes for your trays of water to freeze, as well as the tendency for the center to freeze last, resulting in trapped impurities. Cloudy ice can shatter when you shake it or try to cut it. Clear ice is technically superior and aesthetically pleasing.

## APOTHEKE ACADEMY

The Apotheke Academy features interactive, hands-on mixology and cocktail classes on-site. Participants learn the Apotheke art of crafting medicinal cocktails from one of our expert mixologists. Academy classes are popular for date nights, group parties, company team-building, and client events. Apotheke Academy courses are also available to hire for off-site private events. On-site classes can accommodate up to twenty people, and off-site capacity depends on the specific location. Classes are two hours, and participants craft four unique cocktails.

# ABSINTHE, THE ILLUSTRIOUS GREEN FAIRY

*Dramatic Myths, Belle Époque Glitz, and the Alluring Ritual*

**A**BSINTHE IS A HIGH-PROOF HERBAL SPIRIT MADE FROM wormwood, aniseed, fennel, and other herbs, with a licorice-like flavor from the anise. Also called the green fairy, or *la fée verte*, the drink's green color is attributable to the infused herbs' chlorophyll.

La Belle Époque (1871–1914)—French for "the Beautiful Era"—is the period that brought the world the Moulin Rouge, as well as the Eiffel Tower. Absinthe infiltrated French culture during this sensual and artistic period. We channel the swagger of the Belle Époque on Sunday nights, when we offer the traditional pour, complete with a fairy-adorned absinthe fountain and absinthe cocktails. We offer thirteen different absinthes from the United States, France, and Switzerland.

## Myths, Scandals, and Controversies

No, absinthe doesn't make you hallucinate or go crazy! Wormwood contains a compound called thujone that was believed to be a hallucinogenic. Thujone is a dangerous neurotoxin at large concentrations, but absinthe only has trace amounts of thujone—not nearly enough to cause any toxic effects. Several plants contain thujone, including sage (in a much higher concentration than in wormwood) and tarragon.

Myths about absinthe's effects, which have been thoroughly debunked, range from hallucinations, seizures, and criminal dementia to causing Van Gogh to cut off his ear. Whispers about the dangers of absinthe and the misperception that it is a hallucinogen persist, and have made their way into movies and shows even today.

In a rather random twist of fate, the French wine industry and a pest named phylloxera (*Daktulosphaira vitifoliae*), native to America, helped give rise to absinthe's popularity in France during the famed Belle Époque era. In a kind of reverse Statue of Liberty situation, Americans gifted France with some native grapevines. No one knew until the late 1800s that these vines were infested with phylloxera, since the American grapevines weren't affected by them. European grapes certainly were, and unbeknownst to anyone at the time, that is the reason that Thomas Jefferson's attempts to grow imported French grapes for wine had failed. Phylloxera ravaged France's vineyards and ruined its wine industry in the nineteenth century. Into this void spilled absinthe, much to wine-makers' chagrin, and the rest is history.

The jealous wine industry even tried to blame absinthe for murder. In 1905, Jean Lanfray murdered his wife and kids in rural Switzerland after drinking a small amount of absinthe and copious amounts of white wine and other alcohol throughout the day. This could have been bad for the region that made the wine, so they pinned it on absinthe instead. In the courtroom, a psychiatrist testified that Lanfray suffered from "absinthe madness," which caught on with the public, and the media dubbed the case "The Absinthe Murders" (clearly, sensationalism in the press is not only a recent trend). People do like their drama.

## Medicinal Properties

Absinthe was first marketed as a medicinal elixir for stomach problems and later as a cure-all. It was used to help digestion and to kill intestinal parasites, like roundworms or tapeworms. Wormwood, one of absinthe's main ingredients, has been used to treat digestive problems and kill roundworms for thousands of years. Anise, which gives absinthe its distinct flavor, has also been a staple of medicinal healing manuals for centuries.

Around 1830–1840, absinthe was put in water for French soldiers in Algeria to help protect them from dysentery and other illnesses, and upon their return, they asked for absinthe in the cafes and salons of Paris. Parisian cafes went on to establish a culture of absinthe drinking for the bourgeois class and returning soldiers. The ritual of gathering after work to partake in absinthe gained the nickname "the green hour"—*l'heure verte*—in France.

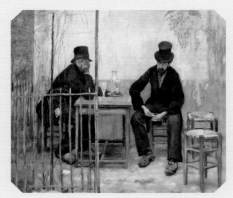

*The Absinthe Drinkers (Les déclassés)* by French Realist painter Jean-François Raffaëlli, 1881.

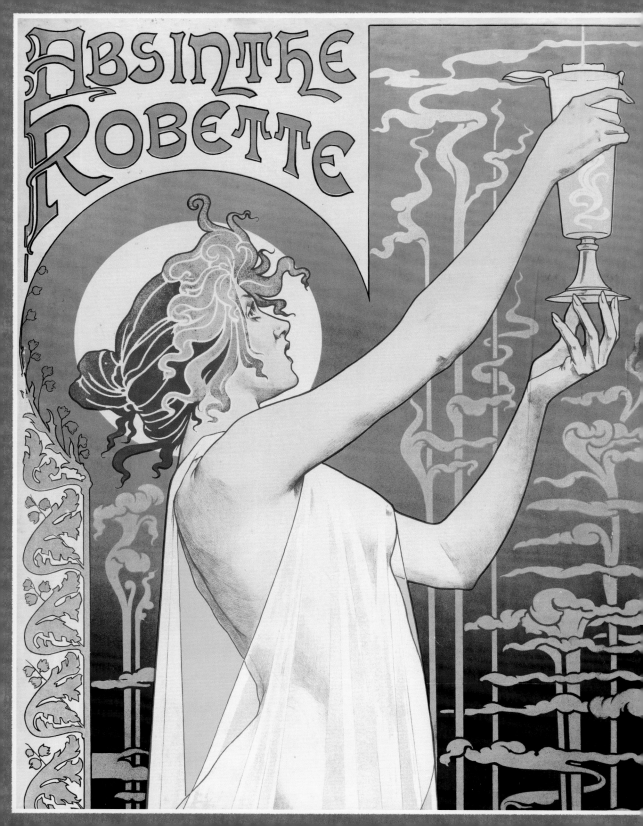

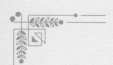

# TRADITIONAL ABSINTHE PREPARATION

*Imbibing absinthe is meant to be a beautiful and even romantic experience. Traditional absinthe preparation is a ceremony of sorts; it gathers drinkers around an absinthe fountain, and the absinthe is poured slowly with an ice-water drip. The louche, the visual spectacle that forms ethereal clouds in the drink as cold water and absinthe dance together, is one of absinthe's most endearing traits. Instructions for the traditional pour follow.*

## Supplies

*Absinthe*
*Absinthe fountain*
*Ice*
*Water*
*Absinthe glass*
*Absinthe spoon*
*Sugar cube*

## Steps

☛ An absinthe fountain lets you control the water drips. These range in style and complexity, from simple to elaborate.

☛ Absinthe glasses often have a demarcation line to help measure the amount of absinthe to pour into it. The water-to-absinthe ratio ranges from 5:1 to 3:1. Put the appropriate amount of absinthe and water in the drip fountain with ice.

☛ Absinthe spoons are distinctive, rather flat, slotted spoons. In the 1800s, sugar came in irregular lumps—not the nice, neat cubes we're used to. So the French invented a spoon that could hold the rocks of sugar.

☛ Some experts view the addition of sugar as optional. But if you'd like to include some, rest the spoon over the glass and place a sugar cube on top. After turning the lever on the fountain, the absinthe will trickle out, drip by drip, through the sugar cube into the glass below.

☛ The *louche* is a fascinating chemical reaction that changes the color of absinthe from pale green to a milky color. It occurs due to characteristics of the essential oils in the plants—they are unstable in alcohol solutions. Adding cold water to the absinthe breaks their chemical bonds, and the oils are set free. At each level of dilution, different flavors will be gradually released.

Belgian artist Privat-Livemont's 1896 *Absinthe Robette* enjoys its association with art nouveau absinthe posters more than a century later—perfectly capturing the whimsical mystique of the green fairy.

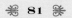

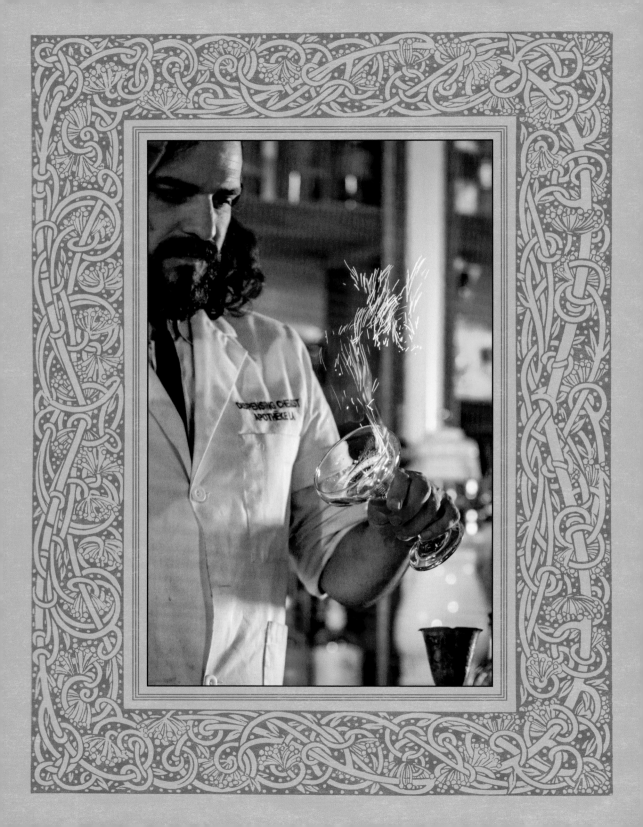

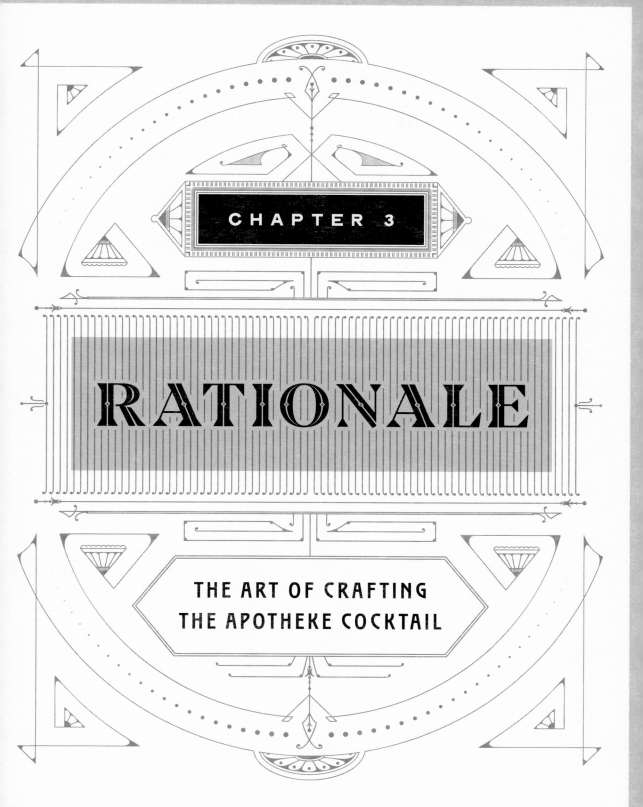

# CHAPTER 3

# RATIONALE

## THE ART OF CRAFTING
## THE APOTHEKE COCKTAIL

**T**HERE IS NO LIMIT TO WHAT CAN BE PUT IN A GLASS. With a respect for and knowledge of the past, we move toward the future and the unlimited possibilities of combinations of liquids and botanicals. Through exploration, creativity, and balance, any visceral sensation can be translated into a libation. Because of this approach, Apotheke has been at the forefront of the modern cocktail frontier, and we have established ourselves as a leader in the plant-based mixology world. Our philosophies and craft continue to push flavor profiles to new heights. From an idea through to execution, the following sections describe the main pillars of our proprietary process.

Flavor is the distinctive taste of a food or drink or an indication of the essential character of something. How you perceive the taste of a food or drink can differ from someone else; grapefruit may be unpleasantly bitter to one person but register as sour to another. The foundation of Apotheke's cocktails is an unclouded collection of balanced natural flavors that excite the palate. To best manipulate and extract flavor, it's important to first understand how we interpret the sensations that direct the palate. Let's break down the science of how our palate registers flavor.

Flavor is an amalgamation of the following complex sensations: taste, smell, touch, and the perception of pain.

## Taste

Taste buds are sensory organs that register chemical inputs. Taste buds are located in the oral cavity, primarily on the tongue, but also line our entire mouth and throat. There are hundreds of taste buds within each papilla, which are the thousands of small bumps on the tongue visible to the naked eye.

## Smell

Olfactory receptors work to register and identify different odors. It is estimated that humans can detect up to 1 trillion distinct smells.

## Touch

The word *astringent* is derived from the Latin *adstringere*, which means "to bind fast." Astringent compounds are the chemicals that shrink or constrict body tissues. This contraction is relayed to the brain. Common astringents include citrus juice, sage, and turmeric.

## Spice

Spiciness is the sensation of pain and irritation that we get from eating pungent or "hot" foods, but it isn't actually detected by our taste buds. Capsaicin, an active component in chili peppers, for example, binds to vanilloid receptors that then transmit a message to our brain that something feels hot.

# TYPES OF TASTE

**H**UMAN TASTE BUDS CAN DETECT FIVE MAIN TASTES: sweet, sour, bitter, salty, and savory (a more fun word for savory is *umami*). These five areas of taste represent the matrix our mixologists use to build their concoctions. The combination of two or more of these distinct elements into one harmonious flow creates a flavor journey. With adequate knowledge of how these taste elements work and their delicate symbiosis, personal creativity can blossom and craft a unique liquid experience.

## Sweet

Although sweetness itself can be used as a prominent flavor profile, it's widely used as an essential balancing technique. Sweet elements can be great allies when incorporating strong ingredients into the imperfections of high-proof alcohol. Sweet notes are also desirable to humans on a biological level. They indicate that herein lie some carbohydrates, which are high in calories and a basic need of the human body. Plants take advantage of our natural instinct to seek out the highest possible calorie intake, so sweet flavors are prevalent in nature. There are many different intensities and varieties of sweetness that we work with. Contrary to what's common for sweet and fruity drinks, we use sweetness more as a balancing and elevating agent rather than a dominant flavor. Sweetness can open the doorway to more exotic flavors and compounds.

## Sour

Sour, much like sweet, can be the star attraction as well as an invaluable team member. Sour taste in nature is mainly connected with different forms of acids. This includes citric, malic, oxalic, propionic, tartaric, and lactic acids. A sour sensation is caused when hydrogen ions are split off by an acid dissolved in a watery

PREVIOUS SPREAD: Nicolas O'Connor, Apotheke mixology director, summons his inner sorcerer as he makes sparkles dance out of the glass.

❦ 85 ❦

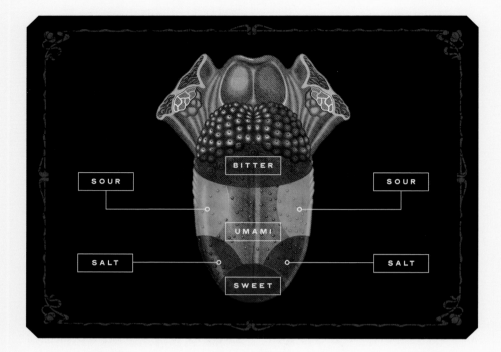

solution. From a chemical point of view, acids can be distinguished by their pH index, which is the activity of protons in a solution. Stronger sour ingredients have a lower pH index, generally between 1 and 3. Weaker sour notes generally have a pH index between 3 and 7. Sweet and sour are yin and yang—opposite realms of the taste spectrum that round out the whole. We see this to be true in our mixology practice. Structuring sour in tandem with sweet creates a baseline canvas upon which other elements can be built. We often start a cocktail with this foundation, as it offers a well-rounded body that provides more control when adding more concentrated taste profiles.

## Bitter

Bitter is an intriguing flavor to highlight, and the distinct taste is plentiful in nature. Along with many animals, we are predisposed to shy away from bitter flavors. Many different species of plants, some of which are poisonous, developed their bitter taste as a defense mechanism (quite clever for non-sentient organisms).

Despite being used for a century, there is open debate in scientific circles on the exact location of these receptors.

Alkaloids, one of plants' bitter-tasting toxins, showed up in plants around the same time that mammals evolved. Thus, our brain jumps right to the panic button when we first taste something bitter. But there is much more to bitter plants than the biological evolutionary background. They offer excellent flavor possibilities and can come with a range of health benefits, including an abundance of antioxidants. Moreover, some cultures view bitter plants and foods as essential to medicine and a healthy diet. In total, there are about thirty-five different proteins in human sensory cells that respond to bitter substances. Bittering agents, or cocktail "bitters," got their start in medicine and have become a dominant component in craft cocktail culture. We implement bitter notes to expand and brighten a cocktail's taste profile.

## Salty

While generally used as an accompanying or finishing ingredient, salinity does contain a variety of other uses. A salty taste is produced by high sodium chloride levels. The salt taste receptor, or epithelial sodium channel, is the simplest receptor found in the mouth. Thus, salt is widely used to elevate other distinct flavors. Just like its culinary use, where an under-use of salt makes a whole dish fall flat, salinity in a cocktail can round out other flavors and make featured ingredients pop. Behind our bar, we use salt and salinity as a chef would.

## Savory/Umami

Savory, also referred to by its Japanese name *umami*, translates to good flavor. This is the most recently acknowledged member of the five basic tastes and the hardest to perceive and define. It is generally described as rich, which can be attributed to the high protein levels. Protein is said to attract and evoke pleasant emotions in most people. It creates a long-lasting, mouthwatering sensation on the tongue. The sensation of umami is due to the detection of the carboxylate anion of glutamate in specialized receptor cells present on the human tongue. Where possible, we like to push the boundaries of conventional taste. Since savory flavors are generally associated with solid foods, incorporating them into liquid form offers a fresh and unexpected experience. Cocktails that showcase a savory bouquet blur the lines between kitchen and bar, where the culinary standard is combined with the cocktail.

# AROMA

**SMELL IS RESPONSIBLE FOR 80 TO 90 PERCENT OF FLAVOR.**
Not only is it our oldest sense, it is also the only one hardwired to the emotion and memory parts of our brain. Smelling with the external nostrils is called orthonasal olfaction; internal smelling at the back of the mouth is called retronasal olfaction. When a smell is registered, the data goes to the brain, which then searches for a match, like a computer database. Think of the last time you had a cold: a stuffy nose dulls flavor perception. The nose picks up volatile compounds in fruits and vegetables—volatile means that they are light enough to jump off their home on the plant and into your nose—and the compounds bind with receptors in the nose. Smell is often overlooked in cocktails, but we know better. Given its scientific significance, we begin the flavor experience with aroma. We finish every cocktail with a thoughtful garnish. Oftentimes the aroma from the garnish is responsible for establishing the full flavor experience.

# TOUCH: ASTRINGENCY

**ASTRINGENCY IS THAT MOUTH-PUCKERING, DRY FEELING WE**
get when we drink a hearty red wine, sip a strong tea, or bite into an unripe fruit. Neither smell nor taste, astringency is a tactile sensation caused by a group of phenolic compounds called tannins. These tannins bond to our saliva's proteins, leading to a clumping effect that removes the usual lubrication that occurs naturally. Astringency does not back down, and it only becomes more pronounced as you continue to consume the tannins.

## APO CANDLES: SETTING THE MOOD AND PRIMING THE SENSES

Aroma doesn't have to stop at the drinks. Given the impact smell has on flavor and mood, we designed custom fragrances from a blend of essential oils and botanicals that accentuate and enhance the flavors in our drinks. We made a unique scent for each of our locations, inspired by their surrounding neighborhoods and respective menus. These all-natural candles are 80 percent soy, 20 percent coconut, and 100 percent captivating.

The LA candle has guaiac wood, also known as palo santo, as one of its base scents (along with fir needle, white birch, amber, rose, and more). Palo santo is an aroma that inspired our drink Pink Panther (page 147)—which uses palo santo–smoked rum.

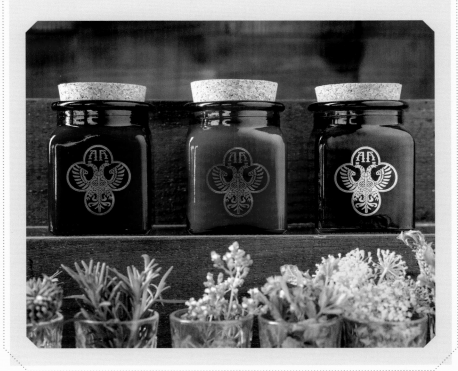

# CREATIVE PROCESS

*Inspiration can find you in every aspect of life. I try to draw from the world that surrounds me in my journeys. Even the visual beauty of a sunset. An idea can hit at any moment.*

—NICOLAS O'CONNOR, *Apotheke Mixology Director*

## Creating Infused Spirits

Infusing liquors involves soaking a botanical ingredient in alcohol for a certain amount of time in order to impart the plant's flavor and aroma to the liquid—and to extract its nutritional benefits.

Using an infused liquor is a great way to elevate your cocktail. It adds complexity, depth, and another layer of flavor. On a practical level, infusing will save you time when it comes to making the drink, and it's a good way to maintain consistency across drinks.

Some flavors aren't easy or appropriate to add toward the end of cocktail construction. Infusing liquors is a way to bypass this. Another gap that infusion can fill: it extracts necessary flavors from botanicals that don't muddle well; this includes vanilla bean and rosemary.

Plants act differently in an infusion situation. The key is to not over-infuse. If you leave certain herbs infusing for too long, the result will be bitter and unappetizing. Basil, cilantro, and other tender green herbs are prime examples of what not to over-infuse. Done right, the liquor will have a hint of the herb or spice's flavor, without the ingredient being overpowering. Done wrong, the liquor will turn a deep, unnatural-looking green, and it will taste very bitter. Watch out for tannin-containing solids, like tea, as they are especially fast in their pivot to unpalatable. But it's easy to avoid the bitter flavor they release after a certain amount of time: put together a small batch first and use this as your test case. Taste the test batch after fifteen minutes, and then every thirty minutes thereafter until you feel the optimal taste has been reached. The moment it tastes right, strain it for use—the infusion is ripe.

The principle of regularly tasting your creation to see if any adjustments are needed applies here as well. Just as apothecaries were known to employ their keenly developed senses to assess the quality of medicinal materials, one must practice using sight, smell, and taste to get the right level of infusion.

## WHAT TO INFUSE: FRUIT, HERBS, SPICES

Your solid ingredient for infusion should be aromatic, colorful, flavorful, and porous. Most plant products have pores and are good candidates for infusing into liquors. It can be useful to increase the surface area of the solid ingredient, exposing more of its pores to the solvent. This could involve chopping, cutting, grinding, or in the case of tea, using loose leaves.

You can use a wide variety of liquors as a base for the infusion, including amazake, bourbon, cachaça, Cognac, gin, Lillet Blanc, mezcal, moonshine, pisco, rum, rye, Scotch, tequila, vodka, and whiskey. Vodka lends itself particularly well to infusions, due to its neutral character. Infused liquors can serve as the main spirit of a cocktail or as a modifier.

Higher proof liquors are the fastest to infuse; lower proof spirits take longer.

You can certainly experiment with the high-tech tools available for infusions (such as the iSi cream whipper for rapid infusions). But it can be done very simply, with no special equipment or techniques: put your solid ingredient in a clean jar (preferably a nonreactive glass or plastic container, with a wide enough mouth to fit in a spoon for stirring) and cover it with the liquor. Seal it tightly and stash it somewhere dark and cool. Taste frequently until it is ready, at which point strain or double strain the mixture, discard the solid, and return the liquor to its original bottle. An exception to this room-temperature preparation is when you have multiple ingredients; store the infusion in the refrigerator if so. Either way, finished infusions can be stored at room temperature or in the refrigerator, depending on how long you plan to keep them.

## Elixirs

Spirit service and house-made elixirs: Our house-made spirits use organic herbs, botanicals, and produce. The infused liquor options include sage and matcha gin and eucalyptus and spirulina tequila. Guests choose two house-made elixirs, and the elixirs are meant to accompany the house-infused spirits.

## Tinctures

Tinctures generally focus on one ingredient instead of a mix of botanical ingredients like bitters. As with bitters, tinctures use a high-proof spirit as the base, which draws out the healing properties of the tinctured ingredient and preserves it. They have long been a fixture in apothecary shops to help treat a wide range of ailments. One of the most unusual tinctures we've created is a deer antler velvet tincture.

## Sweeteners

Common sweeteners include agave (raw blue agave is recommended), honey (as part of a cordial or in an otherwise dissolvable vehicle), sugar, and syrups.

Cordials and liqueurs are critical elements in some cocktails, and they can add sweetness. A cordial is a mixture of a spirit, flavorings, and sugar (usually added at the end). House-made cordials include ancho chili, lavender, and orange (page 227). Liqueurs are spirits that are sweetened and flavored with aromatic botanicals.

## Techniques: Mixing the Magic

### STIRRING

Stirring is reserved for when cocktails call solely for liquor; once you introduce any type of citrus juice or other botanical ingredient to a drink, you steer yourself into the shake lane. Agitating the herbs

induces them to give off more aroma and taste. As such, most of our cocktails are shaken (see pages 74–75 for information about common shaker types).

Stirring is best done with a bar spoon. Keep the back of the spoon in contact with the inside of the glass, which will help you maneuver around ice.

### SHAKING

The purpose of shaking is threefold: to dilute, chill, and add texture in the form of tiny air bubbles. Keep in mind that these little bubbles don't last long, and a shaken cocktail is at its prime immediately after straining. The quality declines every moment it's not consumed. The best ice strategy to achieve a well-rounded result on all three measures is 1¼-inch to 1½-inch solid, square cubes—and remember to remove the surface water from the ice first. For a discussion of ice considerations, see pages 76–77.

Sore arms aren't necessary to get a properly shaken drink—shaking is actually pretty efficient. Our mixologists recommend shaking for a long ten seconds at least. In terms of exact style—if you're asking yourself, *do I have to move the shaker in a clockwise circle, or go up and down?*—you can develop your own. Bartenders have a variety of strategies, angles, and motions; it all comes down to getting the right dilution, chilling, and texture effects rather than exact shaking form. Some of our mixologists

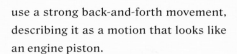

use a strong back-and-forth movement, describing it as a motion that looks like an engine piston.

### DOUBLE STRAINING

To double strain is to strain the contents of a shaker through a Hawthorne strainer into a tea strainer held over the finish glass.

### MUDDLING

Muddling breaks up botanical ingredients and facilitates the release of their flavors and aromas. (Muddling basically "smooshes" the ingredients.) Simply rotate the muddler gently once or twice in the mixing glass to release the plants' essence.

You can use gentle to moderate muddling pressure with herbs. Some people suggest not taking too aggressive a stance with the muddler when you're dealing with herbs, so that they won't release a bitter taste and green color; crushing herbs breaks down their cells and releases chlorophyll. When muddling citrus, you will need to use full force to efficiently extract the oils.

Some botanicals are prime candidates for muddling. Basil, snow peas, and dill react well to being moved around and pounded. Peppercorns require some strong muddling to crush them well. Muddling herbs and vegetables can make for easier and shorter preparation in some recipes. But muddling doesn't apply across the board. Rosemary needs to soak, so we infuse it instead. Vanilla should also be

infused rather than muddled—this is how it gives off its flavor.

### PURÉEING

Puréeing can be done with items that are likely already in your kitchen: a blender, a food processor, or even a high-powered coffee grinder. It's a great way to meld two ingredients before adding them to a drink. Purées are a key component of our cocktails. Over the years, we've puréed a variety of fruits and vegetables, including cactus, cucumber, seaweed, dragon fruit, edamame, shiso, ginger, nectarine, pear, pumpkin, smoked pineapple, strawberry, and tamarind.

### RINSING

Rinsing is generally used with very strong flavors—with the goal of allowing a small hint of the flavor to carry through to the end. The most frequent rinse we use is an absinthe rinse. Pour a small amount of the desired rinsing spirit into the cocktail glass, slowly rotate it to coat the glass, and discard the remaining liquid.

### MISTING

Misting can be done pre- or post-pour. Using a small spray mister or atomizer, misting an aroma over an empty glass is more accurate than the rinsing method, and with none of the waste. You can also mist the top of a cocktail, putting an aromatic finishing touch that reaches your nose immediately. Our most common mist

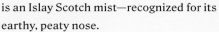
is an Islay Scotch mist—recognized for its earthy, peaty nose.

## RIMMING

Rimming can be used when ingredients complement the flavors of the drink and add something. Arrange the rimming ingredients, which tend to be salt, sugar, or both, on a plate. Use citrus, bitters, or another liquid to wet the upper rim of the glass, and carefully roll it in the rimming solids. Pay attention to how thick you want the rimming line and adjust your roll accordingly. Less is typically better here, as the flavors are concentrated and are the first to hit the palate.

## FAT WASHING

It sounds like it could be labor intensive, but this one is easy. Fat washing is the process of infusing with any ingredient that contains fats. Bacon is a common protein to use with fat washes, but we decided to try something different for our Huntsman cocktail (page 197): duck fat. For a fat wash, pour hot liquid fat into the alcohol and put it in the freezer. The fat will freeze and rise to the top. Remove this cake-like disk of fat. The alcohol is left with the taste of duck or bacon fat (or whatever fat you're using).

## SMOKING

The aroma of smoke incites our appetite and awakens our senses. Smoking is a great way to add some depth and earthy smokiness to a drink. The smokiness of peat is one of the major draws for fans of peaty Scotch. The relationship between humans and fire goes back to our caveman days and associating fire with survival and warmth. Even now, when we smell smoke, it invokes a primal feeling of comfort and sustenance.

Anything porous can absorb smoke and impart a smoky flavor. Hickory-smoked pineapple is a distinctive ingredient in one of our most popular drinks, the Paid Vacation (page 171). We use smoked cloves in the Dead Poet cocktail (page 175). We light the cloves and capture the smoky essence with an upside-down coupe glass. The smoke clings to the surface of the glass. This warm and exotic smell permeates the bar and perks up your senses before you even have the drink in hand.

Alcohol can be smoked just as easily as solid ingredients. See page 147 for the Pink Panther, which uses smoked rum.

## DROPS and DASHES

It's no exaggeration to say that a single drop can make or break a cocktail. The smallest over- or under-pour of concentrated liquids can greatly throw off taste, aroma, or feel. A dropper keeps this in check and gives you control down to the drop, letting you precisely measure and track ingredients.

Using a dropper also gives you control over the specific placement of liquid ingredients. Layers can be created using liquids of different densities. Manipulating these layers not only controls the order in which

*There is a delicate dynamic to Apotheke's atmosphere. Taste, touch, sight, sound, and smell work in harmony to create environments where our customers experience a visceral sense of emotion, have meaningful conversations, and grow relationships.*

—CHRISTOPHER TIERNEY, *Apotheke Founder and Designer*

ingredients register on the palate but can create incredibly unique visual aesthetics.

## Aesthetics

Sight is one of the key senses humans have to seek and sort their food options. One reason that aesthetics matter, and why we're drawn to vibrant-looking foods and drinks, may stem from the fact that deeper-colored fruits and vegetables are healthier. With more sunlight, the leaf needs to produce more antioxidants and pigments, giving it a darker hue, richer skin, beneficial carotenoids, and phenolic compounds.

The psychological connection between taste and visual appeal is strong: a drink's aesthetics can trick your mind into liking it. This is one of our rationales behind harnessing the naturally vibrant beauty of fresh produce to create a very appetizing aesthetic.

Our propensity to enjoy or notice things based on their initial visual appearance is hardwired into our brains. A famous study from 2001 by Frédéric Brochet illustrates

this well. Enology students were given white and red wines and asked to describe their flavors. They responded by giving the usual flavor characteristics of each. Then, the researchers colored the same white wines with red food dye (and tested to ensure that the dye did not affect the flavor), and gave the subjects the white wines next to the "red" wines. Almost all of the participants described the dyed white wines with red wine olfactory and taste characteristics. The sight of red wine primed their brains for a certain experience.

### GARNISHES

Garnishes are sometimes added solely to be pretty and decorative—playing on the hardwired link between sight and the taste buds. But they also serve an important olfactory purpose, imparting a subtle taste that adds to the balance of the flavors. All of our garnishes are intended to be visually enticing and aroma directed, and—except for a select few that are so cool they're worth being inedible—they are 100 percent edible.

# APO BITTERS WITH BENEFITS

*Apotheke's Proprietary Functional Formulas*

**T**HE EXPERT MIXOLOGISTS BEHIND THE BAR AT APOTHEKE have been using proprietary bitter blends since the first location in NYC opened its doors more than a decade ago. And just like everything else you'll find at Apotheke, our bitters have been constantly evolving toward the ideal link between ancient plant knowledge and today's best plant science–based infusions. Meticulously developed with the help of some of today's best herbalists and inspired by humanity's connection to plants, APO™- BITTERS with BENEFITS™ provide plant-based function while also delivering flavor-enhancing profiles for cocktails, teas, sodas, and other beverages.

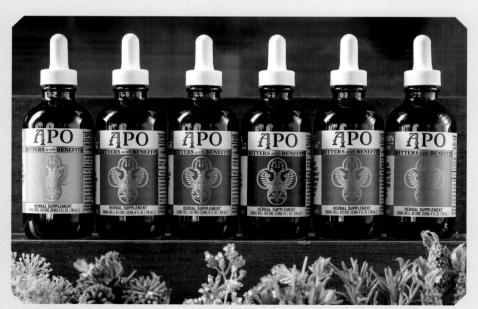

## Illuminate

TASTING NOTES: *Earth, Celery, Savory*

APO ILLUMINATE encourages healthy skin and hair growth and improves circulation by reducing impurities in the bloodstream, while a powerful mix of antioxidants and adaptogens help prevent aging.

## Rejuvenation

TASTING NOTES: *Oak, Floral, Bright*

APO REJUVENATION encourages healthy liver function while promoting cellular repair, easing inflammation, and alleviating common symptoms of a hangover.

## Digestion

TASTING NOTES: *Leaf, Menthol, Pepper*

APO DIGESTION is formulated to encourage effective digestion by relaxing the gastrointestinal tract, stimulating digestive secretions, and restoring balance throughout the GI while cooling and calming discomfort.

## Cerebral

TASTING NOTES: *Fruit, Sweet, Herbaceous*

APO CEREBRAL is a powerful formulation of phytonutrients and nootropics that aid in increasing concentration, help protect and repair neurons, and help boost overall cognitive performance.

## Libido

TASTING NOTES: *Warm, Citric, Robust*

APO LIBIDO is a combination of dynamic adaptogens and potent aphrodisiacs that stimulate adrenal glands, elevate mood, and boost energy while increasing stamina and sexual desire.

## Immunity

TASTING NOTES: *Shroom, Coco, Rich*

APO IMMUNITY is a robust combination of powerful immune-boosting herbs, adaptogens, and medicinal mushrooms that support overall health and wellness while helping to restore and strengthen the body's defense system.

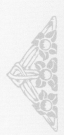
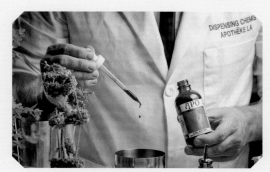
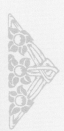

# PART II

---

# THE FORMULAS

## APOTHEKE'S COCKTAILS

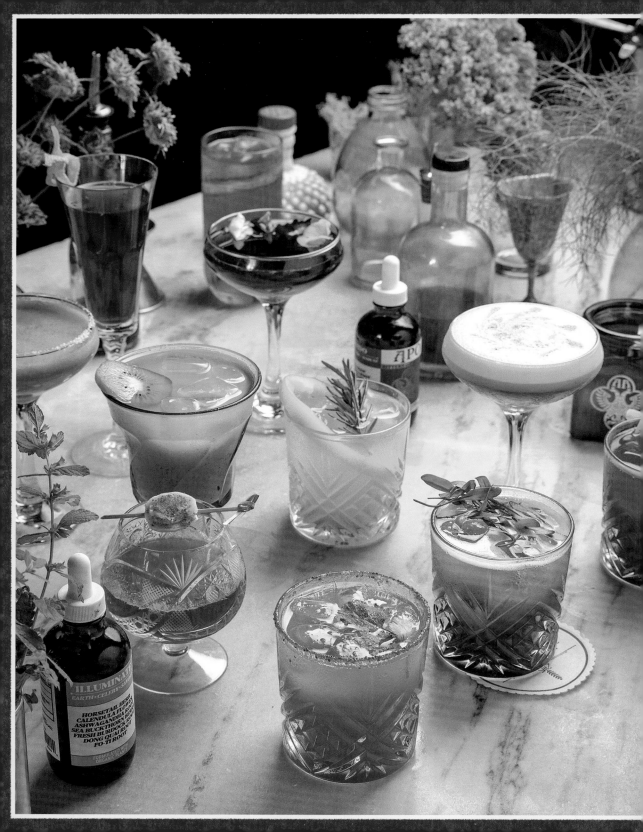

**O**UR COCKTAIL FORMULAS ARE ARRANGED IN SIX categories, based on their ingredients and occasionally the base spirit they use:

# HEALTH & BEAUTY

# APHRODISIACS

# STRESS RELIEVERS

# STIMULANTS

# PAINKILLERS

# EUPHORICS

These categories naturally have overlaps; many herbs have a wide array of healing properties. Feeling healthy, for example, is itself an aphrodisiac. Ashwagandha root, an ingredient in our APO Illuminate Bitters, has aphrodisiac, painkilling, stress-relieving, stimulating, and overall health properties.

All recipes serve one. In fact, our mixologists advocate for making medicinal cocktails one at a time instead of in batches, even if you're making drinks for a party of friends. They reveal that it's easier to control the portions and allows you to pour care into each drink. We hope that reading and making these drinks will connect you to the past, invigorate the present, and use techniques and plant science that illuminate the future. And even if they're not physically present with you, they also connect you to a solidly established global community of cocktail enthusiasts, herbalists, and lovers of plants.

At the end of the formula section is a compendium (pages 226–236) that provides detailed recipes for homemade ingredients.

> *"The 'Cocktail' is a modern invention, and is generally used on fishing and other sporting parties, although some patients insist that it is good in the morning as a tonic."*
> —JERRY THOMAS, *How to Mix Drinks: Or, A Bon-vivant's Companion,*
> also known as *The Bar-Tender's Guide (1862)*

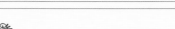

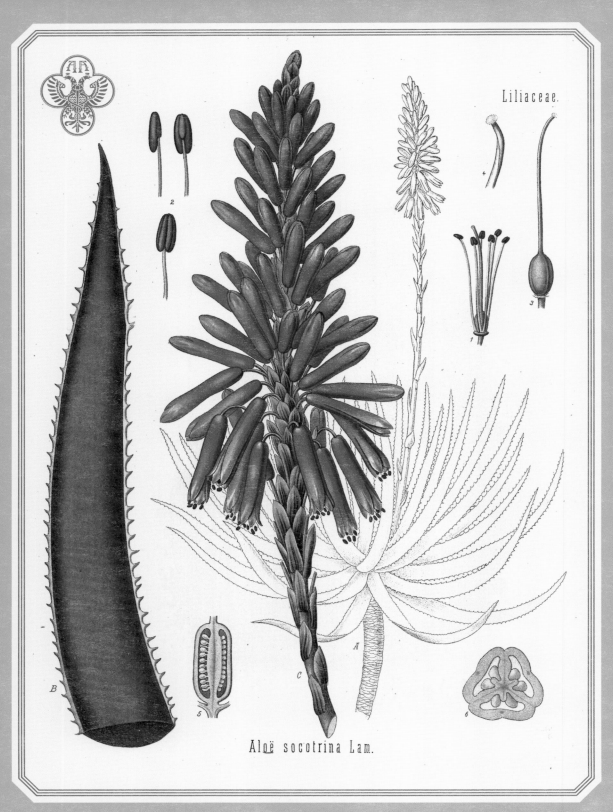

Liliaceae.

Aloë socotrina Lam.

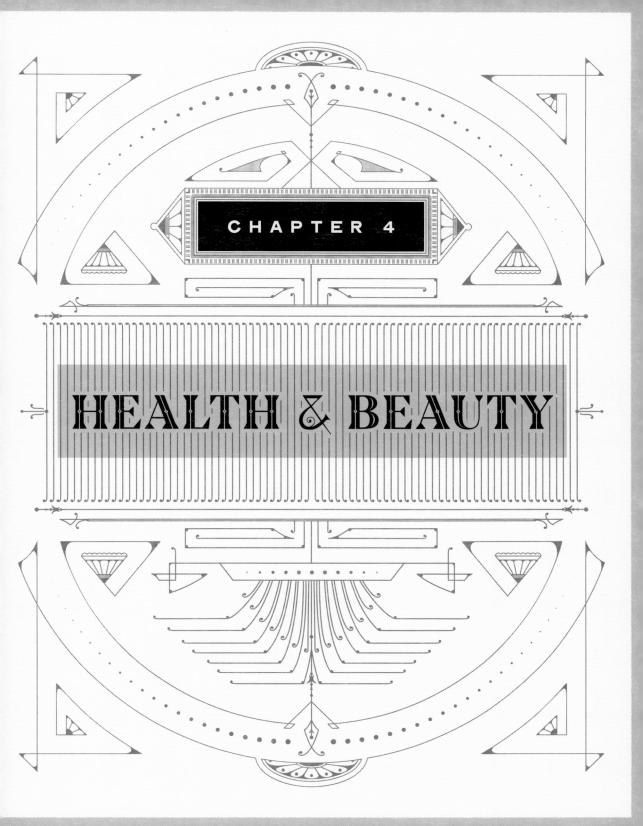

CHAPTER 4

# HEALTH & BEAUTY

THIS COLLECTION OF RECIPES IS DESIGNED FROM SOME of nature's most powerful healers and inspired by natural ingredients containing a multitude of vitamins, minerals, antioxidants, anti-inflammatory compounds, digestive aids, and immunity boosters. Many of the plants in the following recipes have been used for hundreds—or even thousands—of years to rejuvenate the body and aid in overall health. These formulas draw on ingredients that offer a variety of health benefits and are commonly used in skincare, circulatory, and rejuvenating medical processes. These formulas will make you feel good, inside and out.

## Traits of Ingredients in This Chapter

One of the lesser known fruits highlighted in this section, the Cape gooseberry, has a variety of health benefits and contains more antioxidants than broccoli or apples.

Kale is a modern super green. Unfairly relegated to garnish status in the 1990s, it has enjoyed a resurgence in popularity due to its major health benefits. Kale juice works well for enhancing skin and hair health because it's a rich source of vitamin C. The Kale in Comparison (page 113) has become a best seller.

Kiwi: Step aside, oranges and bananas. We often associate oranges with vitamin C and think of bananas as a top source of potassium, but kiwis have more vitamin C than oranges and more potassium than bananas. Kiwis are packed with antioxidants, including vitamin E, polyphenols, and flavonoids. Studies have demonstrated positive impacts of these compounds on lipid profiles and HDL (good cholesterol).

## Stomach Health and Digestion

Having a healthy gut matters. Studies show that the diversity of gut microbes diminishes as people and animals get older. But for the first time, scientists have demonstrated a link between microbiomes and lifespan. A 2017 experiment on fish had striking results: transplanting young gut microbiomes into an older host improved longevity.

Many of the ancient ingredients used in medicinal cocktails have been used for various digestive maladies over the course of thousands of years. If you comb through ancient medical texts and medieval herbals, digestive ailments come up again and again. One of our APO Bitters with Benefits™ is designed for digestive health.

Sure, digestion can easily be overlooked—heart and brain health seem to get a lot of the airtime—but it's critical for how your body feels all day, every day. A healthy digestive system equals a healthy system overall.

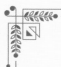
## Spirit Notes

Gin lends itself well to this category, as it's already jam-packed with botanicals from the distilling process. Add more layers to that, and you have a nuanced, herbal formula for rejuvenation. In this section, we balance a diverse range of health benefits with specific flavor profiles to liquify beautiful health.

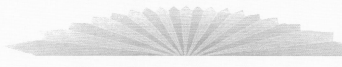

**FEATURED HEALTH & BEAUTY BOTANICALS**

## ALOE VERA

## GOOSEBERRY

## KALE

## POMEGRANATE

## THYME

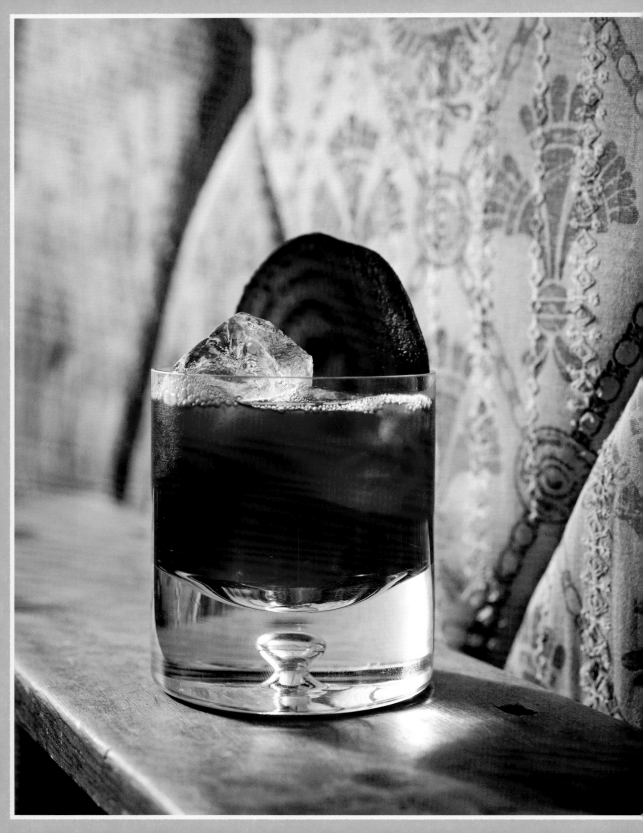

# TAINTED LOVE

*The Tainted Love is a unique blend of flavors. Beet-Infused Gin is paired with Pomegranate Shrub, which utilizes balsamic vinegar to balance out the sweetness of the fruit and sugar. Adding a bit of port wine creates a very rounded, rich cocktail, reminiscent of a Negroni—yet altogether different.*

## FORMULA

2 ounces Beet-Infused Gin *(page 232)*

1 ounce Pomegranate Shrub
*(page 228)*

¾ ounce ruby port wine

½ ounce Sour Mix *(page 227)*

3 dashes Peychaud's Bitters

Garnish beet slice

## TOOLS

Jigger

Shaker

Hawthorne strainer

Rocks glass

## EXECUTION

**Add all of the measured ingredients and ice to a shaker. Shake vigorously.
Strain into a rocks glass with fresh ice. Garnish with a beet slice.**

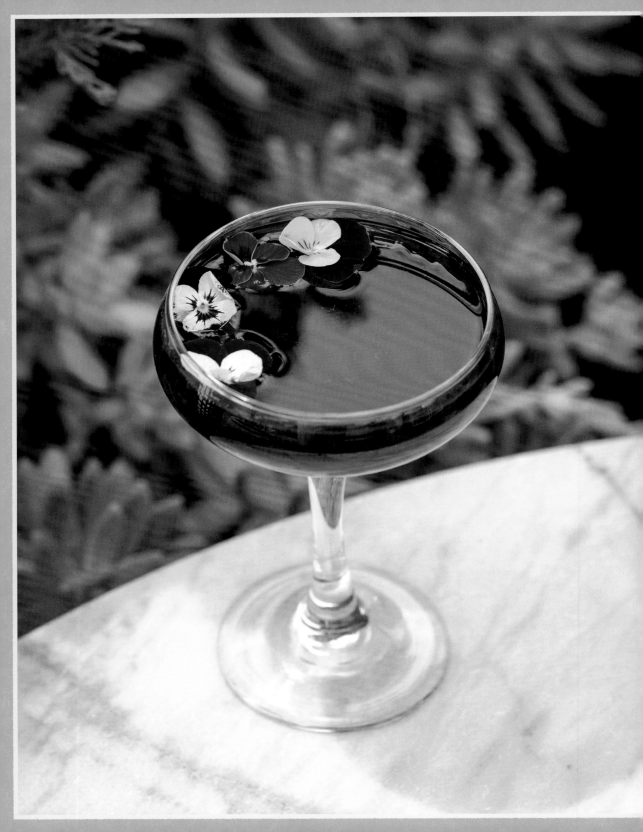

# • QUEEN OF SPADES •

*Don't let the black color fool you: this bright cocktail mixes fresh cucumber and aloe with a pop of bubbles fit for royalty. It is playful yet sophisticated, fruity yet dry, light yet dark. May the reign of this queen be long, delicious, and vain.*

## FORMULA

2 cucumber slices, each ¼ inch thick

2 ounces Activated Charcoal–Infused Vodka *(page 232)*

1 ounce aloe vera juice

½ ounce lime juice

½ ounce Simple Syrup *(page 226)*

1 ounce Champagne

Garnish edible violas

## TOOLS

Shaker

Muddler

Jigger

Lemon squeezer

Hawthorne strainer

Tea strainer

Coupe glass

## EXECUTION

Place the cucumber slices in a shaker. Muddle lightly to break up the cucumbers. Add the vodka, aloe vera and lime juices, Simple Syrup, and ice to the shaker. Shake vigorously. Pour the Champagne into a coupe glass. Double strain (see page 93) the contents of the shaker into the coupe glass. Strain slowly so as not to overexcite the Champagne. Garnish with a few edible violas on top of the cocktail.

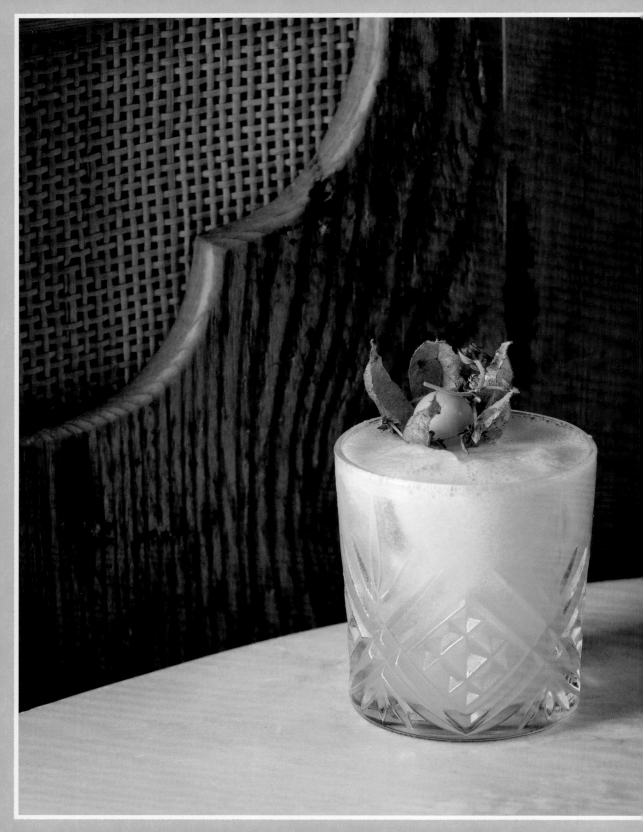

# GOOD FOR THE GANDER

*It is said that what's good for the goose is good for the gander. This tropics-inspired cocktail combines bright Cape gooseberries and cantaloupe to fortify the flavor of the banana, all bonded together with rum and a hint of thyme.*

## FORMULA

2 Cape gooseberries, husked

2 ounces Thyme-Infused Rum
*(page 234)*

1 ounce Cantaloupe-Banana Purée
*(page 229)*

¾ ounce lime juice

½ ounce Simple Syrup *(page 226)*

2 cc APO Illuminate Bitters
*(recommended)*

Garnish gooseberry and thyme

## TOOLS

Shaker

Muddler

Jigger

Lemon squeezer

Hawthorne strainer

Rocks glass

## EXECUTION

Place the gooseberries in a shaker. Muddle just enough to break the skins of the gooseberries. Add all measured ingredients and ice to the shaker. Shake vigorously. Strain the contents into a rocks glass over fresh ice. Garnish with a husked gooseberry and a sprig of thyme on the top of the cocktail.

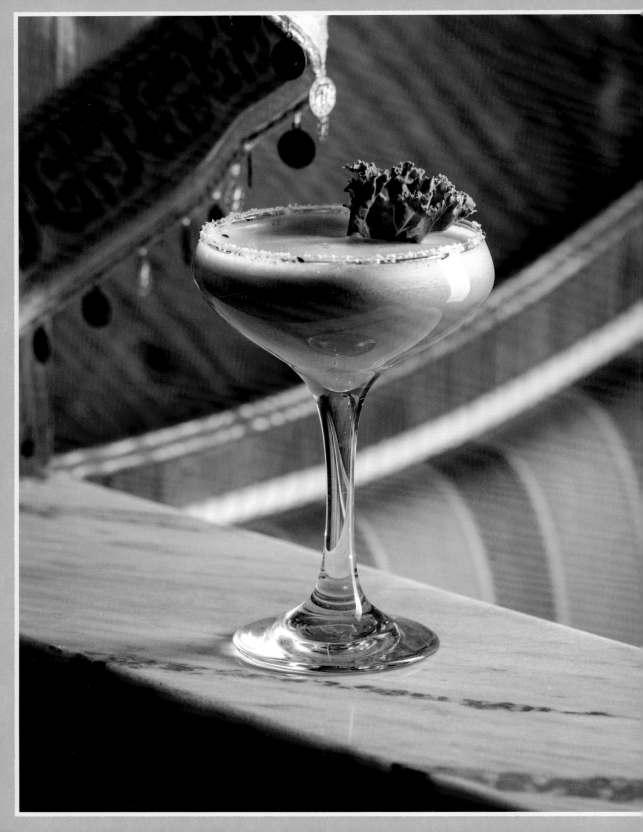

# • KALE IN COMPARISON •

*Earthy, bitter kale, sweet pineapple, sour lime, spicy ginger, and savory house-made Sesame and Anise Sea Salt all fuse together to create a symmetry of flavor. Even with such bold flavors, it's surprisingly compact.*

## FORMULA

2 ounces quinoa vodka

1 ounce Kale-Pineapple Purée
*(page 230)*

¼ ounce Ginger Water *(page 226)*

¾ ounce lime juice

½ ounce Simple Syrup *(page 226)*

2 cc APO Cerebral Bitters
*(recommended)*

Wedge blood orange or other
citrus fruit

Rim Sesame and Anise Sea Salt
*(page 236)*

Garnish kale

## TOOLS

Shaker

Jigger

Lemon squeezer

Hawthorne strainer

Coupe glass

## EXECUTION

Place all of the measured ingredients into a shaker with ice. Shake vigorously. Rub the rim of a coupe glass with a wedge of blood orange. Dip the coupe glass in Sesame and Anise Sea Salt, creating an even line of salt on the rim. Strain the contents of the shaker into the coupe glass. Garnish with a torn piece of fresh kale.

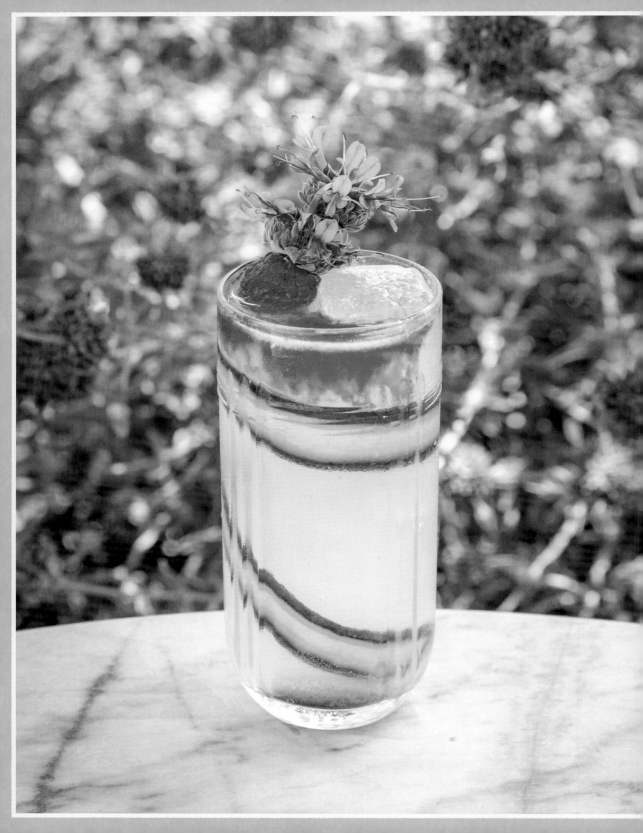

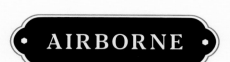

# · AIRBORNE ·

CREATED EXCLUSIVELY FOR THIS BOOK

*Packed with almost every hydrating and uplifting ingredient one can find, it glides onto the palate like a cloud, making its juicy and herbaceous presence known.*

## FORMULA

2 cucumber slices, each ¼ inch thick

1½ ounces Milk Thistle–Infused Vodka *(page 234)*

½ ounce coconut water

¾ ounce aloe vera juice

¾ ounce Meyer lemon juice

½ ounce store-bought maple water

¼ ounce Ginger Water *(page 226)*

½ teaspoon probiotics

Topped with club soda and beet juice

Garnish with raspberries, sage flower, and cucumber ribbon

## TOOLS

Muddler

Shaker

Jigger

Hawthorne strainer

Collins glass

## EXECUTION

Muddle the cucumber slices in a shaker. Add ice and all of the measured ingredients to the shaker. Shake vigorously. Add club soda and beet juice to the shaker. Strain ingredients into a Collins glass with fresh ice and garnish.

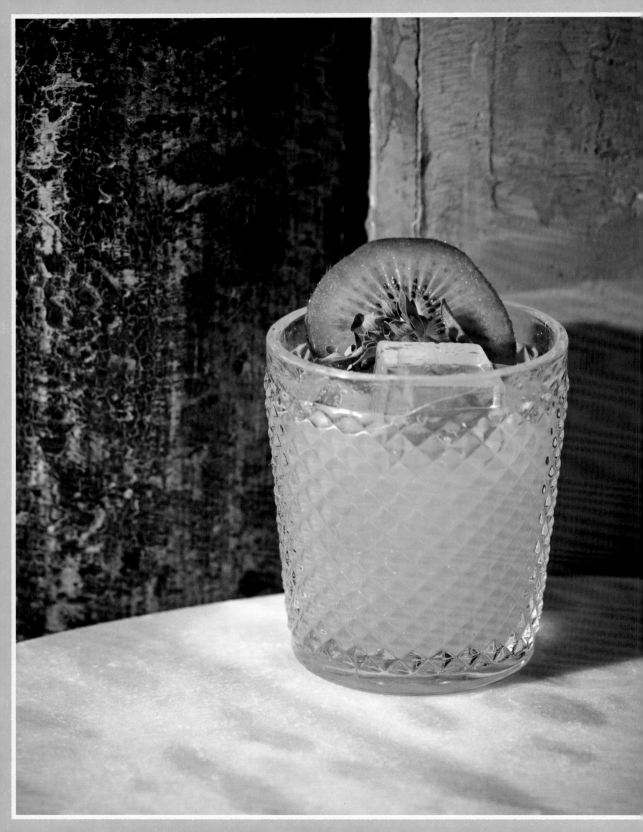

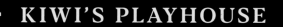

# • KIWI'S PLAYHOUSE •

*Fennel and marjoram, which are great to have in your herbal arsenal, have long histories of healing. This creation is also a great way to explore a couple of less-common spirits from Brazil and Korea, respectively: cachaça and soju (a clear distilled beverage).*

### FORMULA

Kiwi slice

1 stalk fresh fennel

Pinch marjoram

1½ ounces cachaça

1 ounce soju

½ ounce lime juice

Dash agave

Garnish kiwi slice and marjoram

### TOOLS

Muddler

Shaker

Jigger

Lemon squeezer

Hawthorne strainer

Tea strainer

Rocks glass

### EXECUTION

Muddle the kiwi, fennel, and marjoram in a shaker. Add the measured ingredients and ice to the shaker and shake vigorously. Double strain into a rocks glass with fresh ice. Garnish with a kiwi slice and a sprig of marjoram.

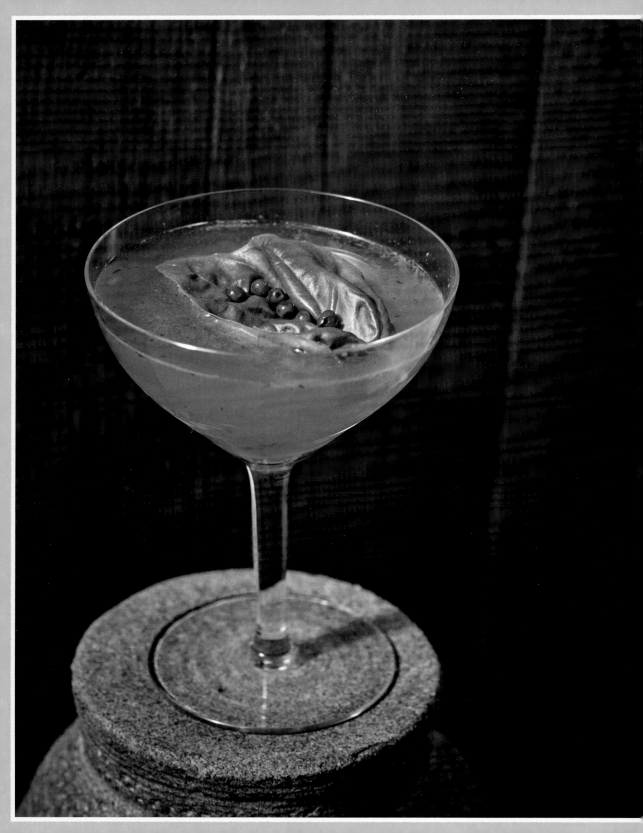

# • STOLEN FROM EDEN •

*This vegetable-packed concoction looks the part, with a beautiful green color reminiscent of a lush, grassy meadow and verdant plants. Gin is the perfect base for the savory ingredients. The power and efficiency of muddling is on full display here; the preparation of the drink is quick and simple due to the ease with which snow peas and basil are muddled.*

## FORMULA

3 snow peas

3 basil leaves

Sprig dill

Bar spoon pink and black
peppercorns

2 ounces gin

¾ ounce Sour Mix *(page 227)*

Garnish basil leaf and pink
peppercorns

## TOOLS

Muddler

Shaker

Jigger

Hawthorne strainer

Tea strainer

Coupe glass

## EXECUTION

Muddle the snow peas, basil, dill, and peppercorns in a shaker. Add the gin, Sour Mix, and ice to the shaker and shake vigorously. Double strain into a coupe glass. Garnish with a basil leaf and pink peppercorns.

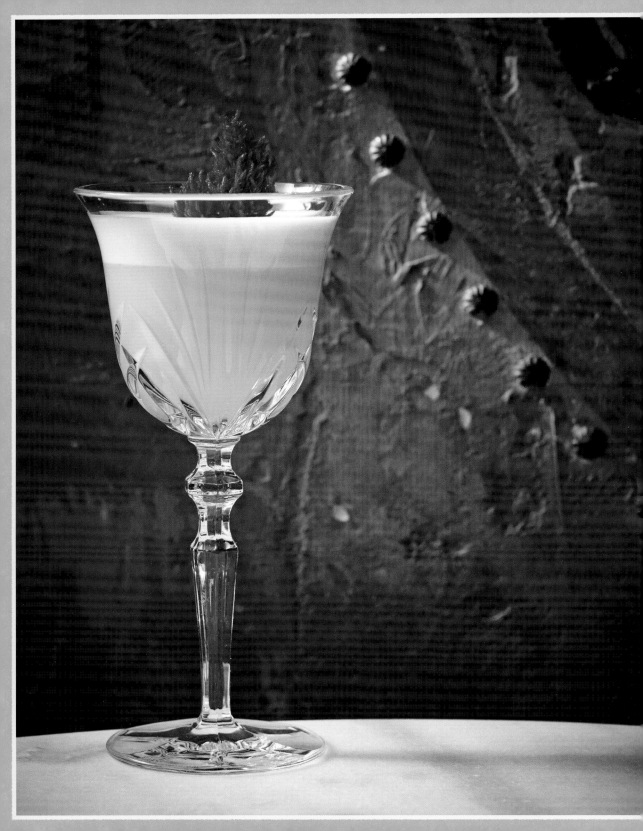

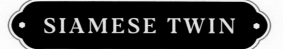

# • SIAMESE TWIN •

*We drew inspiration from our home base in Chinatown and from traditional Japanese ingredients to create this exotic cocktail. It has one of our favorite garnishes: a deep maroon Firestix flower, which is part of the amaranth plant.*

## FORMULA

2 ounces Jasmine Tea and Sake–Infused Vodka *(page 233)*

1 ounce Shiso–Taro Root Purée *(page 231)*

½ ounce Ginger Mix *(page 226)*

¾ ounce Sour Mix *(page 227)*

½ ounce egg white

Garnish Firestix

## TOOLS

Shaker

Jigger

Hawthorne strainer

White wine glass

## EXECUTION

**Combine all of the measured ingredients in a shaker and dry shake (without ice). Add ice and shake vigorously. Strain into a white wine glass and garnish with a Firestix flower.**

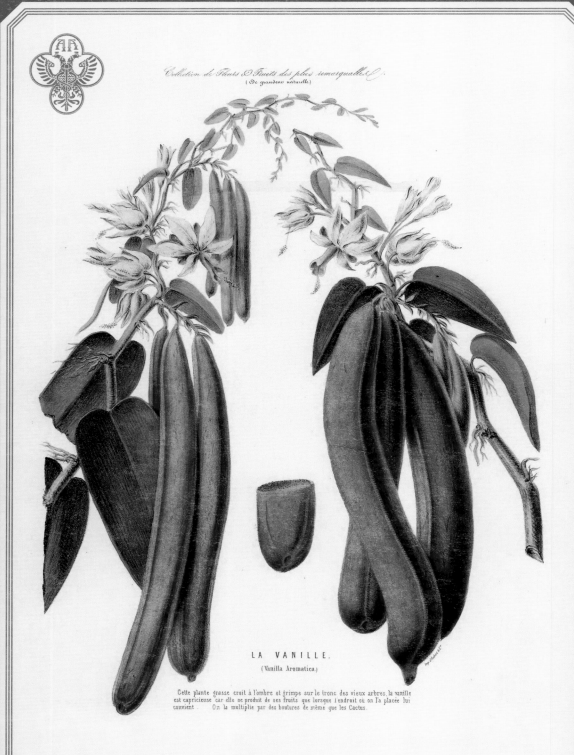

LA VANILLE.

(Vanilla Aromatica.)

Cette plante grasse croit à l'ombre et grimpe sur le tronc des vieux arbres, la vanille
est capricieuse car elle ne produit de ses fruits que lorsque l'endroit où on l'a placée lui
convient.   On la multiplie par des boutures de même que les Cactus.

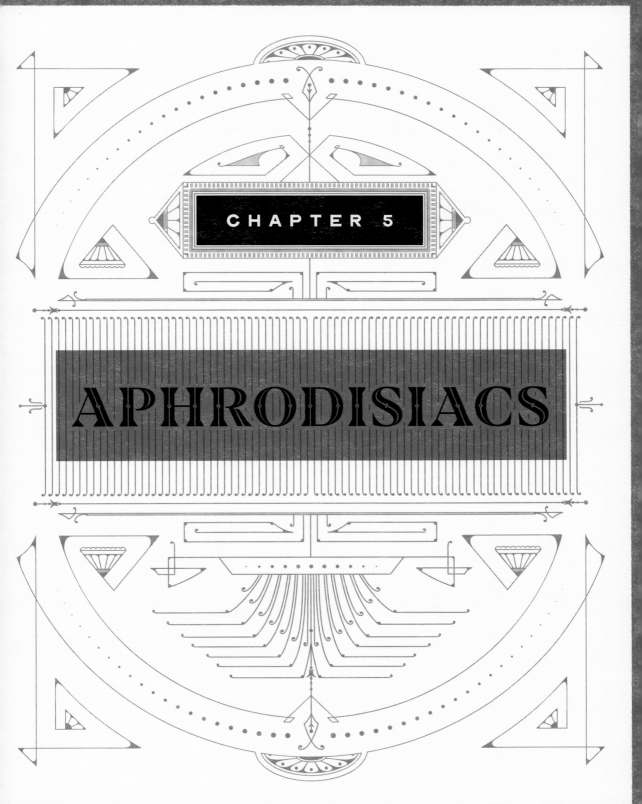

# CHAPTER 5

# APHRODISIACS

# H
**UMANS HAVE LONG SOUGHT TO HARNESS THE SEXUAL**
healing of plants and have (rather arbitrarily) ascribed all sorts of sex-granting powers to everything from oysters to strawberries. During the eighteenth century, aphrodisiac drinks were eccentric yet common, usually sold in hand-painted bottles from apothecary shops.

Several plants that have aphrodisiac effects are included in our selection. We like to think that drinks can be aphrodisiacs simply due to their appearance—as pretty cocktails stimulate the senses and awaken desires.

Pharmacies in nineteenth-century New Orleans sold voodoo potions and powders, in addition to more traditional remedies. The Creoles' unusual blend of cultures—African, French, Native American, and Spanish—enabled voodoo to touch more parts of society than it normally would otherwise. While voodoo wasn't universally accepted, adherents and curious upper-class members would still anonymously buy love and luck potions "under-the-counter," with a numbering system for discretion, at their local pharmacies (which is where the song "Love Potion #9" gets its name). The New Orleans Pharmacy Museum, housed in the former apothecary of Louis Dufilho, contains these voodoo relics alongside other antique medical ephemera that capture the imagination.

An earlier and more bizarre example of love potions comes from a European period where alcoholic medicinal cordials were gaining popularity as stand-alone drinks. In 1447, church authorities censured a woman named Giovanna of San Ambroglio in Florence for going too far in her quest for aphrodisiacs: she dug up skulls in a nearby graveyard and created a powder from them, mixed the powder with wine, and distilled what she called a love potion.

## Traits of Ingredients in This Chapter

The sexual lives of strawberries are surprisingly interesting. In 1712, a French spy brought back a Chilean strawberry. The Chilean strawberry fascinated him, and a bunch of the plants joined him on the ship home. The lone strawberry standing at the end of the voyage ended up being sterile. Unbeknownst to him, these strawberries can be bisexual, female, or male, and he had chosen all females.

Saffron is the most expensive spice in the world (followed by vanilla) due to several factors, including the fact that it's sterile (and thought to be a mutant) and it takes four thousand flowers to make a mere ounce of saffron. Saffron has long been prized for its medicinal qualities. Picrocrocin gives saffron its bitterness and several of its medicinal benefits; studies have found tumor-suppressing and free-radical-scavenging effects, and it helps with digestion. An ancient remedy, it has been used in Ayurvedic medicine for thousands of years, and archaeologists found saffron residue in drinking vessels in King Midas's tomb.

Star anise, the fruit of a small Chinese evergreen tree, is used in traditional Chinese medicine to stimulate circulation. Although unrelated to aniseed, both have a unique licorice flavor. Star anise contains estrogenic compounds (female hormones), which have been reported to induce similar libido-increasing effects as testosterone. The seeds are an excellent source of minerals like iron, magnesium, calcium, manganese, zinc, potassium, and copper.

## Spirit Notes

Vodka is an effective base spirit for aphrodisiac ingredients, due to its neutral character. The ingredients run the gamut in terms of their flavor profiles. Champagne and Cognac also play well as aphrodisiacs.

## FEATURED APHRODISIAC BOTANICALS

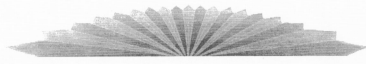

# HORNY GOAT WEED

# MACA ROOT

# SAFFRON

# STAR ANISE

# VANILLA

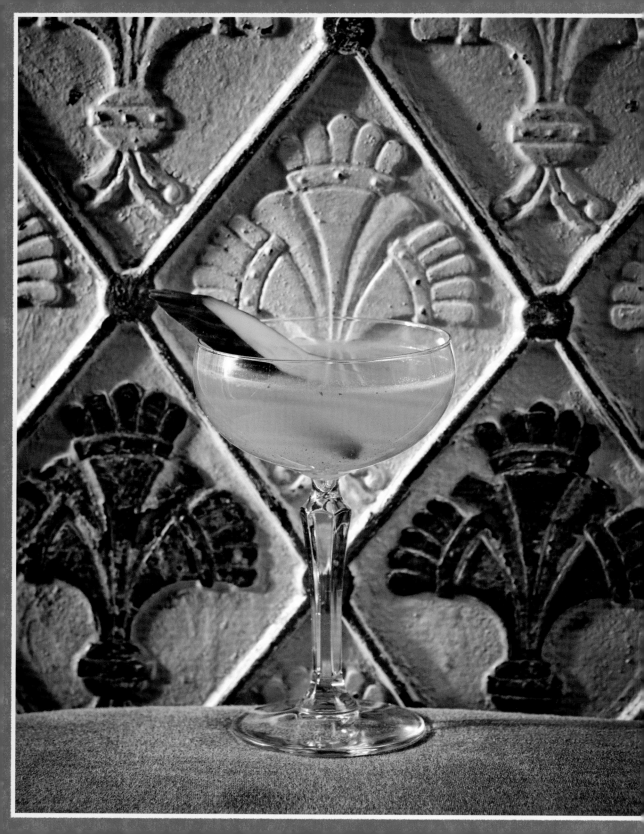

# • DEAL CLOSER •

*Cucumber and mint are a classic combination for a light, refreshing summer respite. As the legend goes, horny goat weed tea is an ancient Chinese fermented black aphrodisiac. We source horny goat weed tea from a local Chinatown tea shop, but it can be purchased online from a variety of retailers. This tea provides a backdrop to properly showcase the more exciting flavors of cucumber and mint. The vanilla Cognac comes in at the end, providing a satisfying aftertaste to wrap up one of our most popular cocktails on the menu.*

### FORMULA

3 cucumber wheels, each ¼ inch thick

Pinch mint leaves

2 ounces vodka

1 ounce horny goat weed tea

1 ounce Sour Mix *(page 227)*

Dash Vanilla-Infused Cognac *(page 234)*

1 cc APO Libido Bitters *(recommended)*

Garnish with bias-cut cucumber

### TOOLS

Muddler

Shaker

Jigger

Hawthorne strainer

Coupe glass

### EXECUTION

**Muddle the cucumber wheels and mint in a shaker. Add the measured ingredients with ice and shake vigorously. Strain into a coupe glass. Garnish with the cucumber surfboard.**

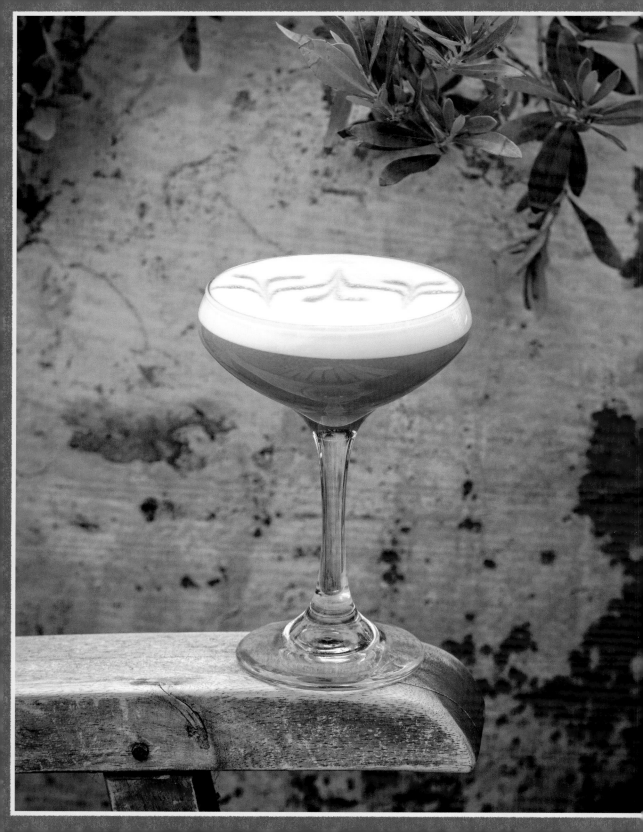

# • HOLLYWOOD ANTOINETTE •

*As bright, bold, and beautiful as a Hollywood starlet, yet as poised, delicate, and sophisticated as French royalty. Strawberry and prickly pear take center stage in this variation on a pisco sour. Its presentation will grab a hold of you; its performance will take you on a ride.*

## FORMULA

2 strawberries

2 ounces pisco

1 ounce Prickly Pear Purée *(page 231)*

½ ounce lime juice

½ ounce Simple Syrup *(page 226)*

½ ounce egg white

2 cc APO Libido Bitters
*(recommended)*

Garnish Angostura bitters

## TOOLS

Muddler

Shaker

Jigger

Lemon squeezer

Hawthorne strainer

Coupe glass

Bitters dropper

## EXECUTION

Muddle the strawberries in a shaker. Add the measured ingredients and dry shake (without ice). Add ice and shake vigorously. Slowly strain into a coupe glass. Garnish by using a dropper to apply the Angostura bitters to the foam on top of the coupe glass.

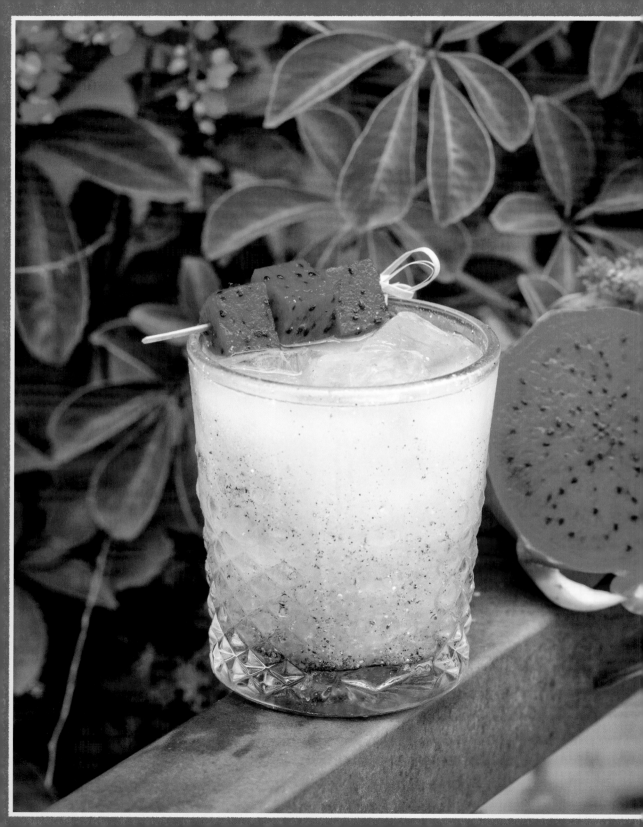

# • FORLORN DRAGON •

*There's nothing sad about the Forlorn Dragon. The mix of tart blueberries with fresh and earthy blended dragon fruit soars above the rich and complex Cognac and Jamaican rum base. An adventurous endeavor indeed.*

## FORMULA

1 ounce Cognac

1 ounce Jamaican rum

1 ounce Blueberry–Dragon Fruit Purée *(page 229)*

½ ounce orgeat syrup *(see note)*

½ ounce lime juice

Garnish dragon fruit cubes and pinch garam masala

## TOOLS

Jigger

Lemon squeezer

Shaker

Hawthorne strainer

Rocks glass

## EXECUTION

**Add the the measured ingredients to a shaker with ice. Shake vigorously. Strain the ingredients into a rocks glass with fresh ice. Garnish with dragon fruit cubes. Sprinkle a pinch of garam masala over the top.**

NOTE: Orgeat is a sweet syrup made from almonds, sugar, and rose or orange flower water and can be purchased online or at well-stocked liquor stores.

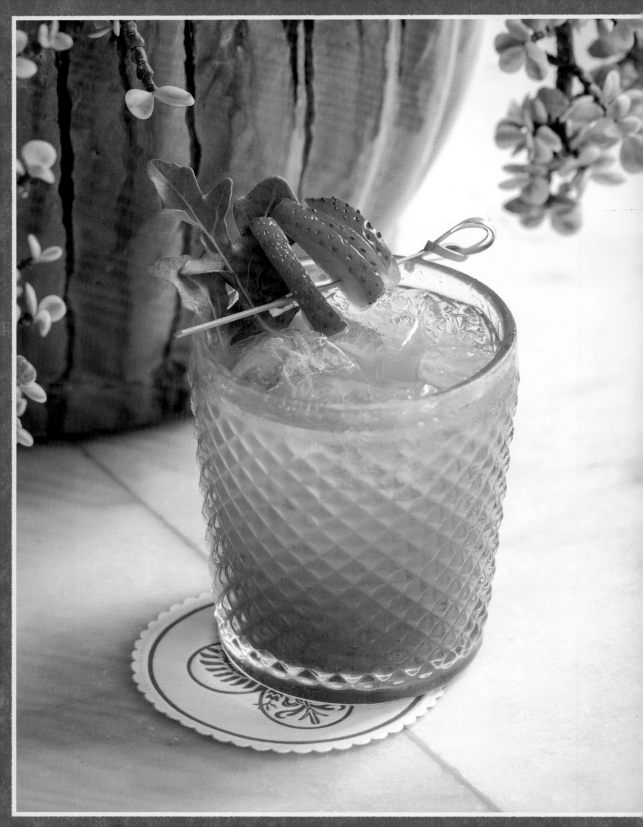

# • HAND IN HAND •

CREATED EXCLUSIVELY FOR THIS BOOK

*Flavor and health working side by side, blending ingredients from all areas of the palate. Familiar yet exotic, complex but clean, nutritious and great tasting. As with ancient traditions of drinking aquavit—the water of life—join with the Hand in Hand and surrender to the romance.*

## FORMULA

1 ounce Maca-Infused Rum *(page 234)*

1 ounce aquavit

1 ounce Strawberry, Watermelon, and Arugula Purée *(page 231)*

½ ounce red ginseng tea

¾ ounce lime juice

½ ounce Simple Syrup *(page 226)*

Garnish strawberry and arugula

## TOOLS

Jigger

Shaker

Hawthorne strainer

Rocks glass

## EXECUTION

Add all of the measured ingredients to a shaker with ice. Shake vigorously. Strain the shaker into a rocks glass over fresh ice. Garnish with strawberry and arugula.

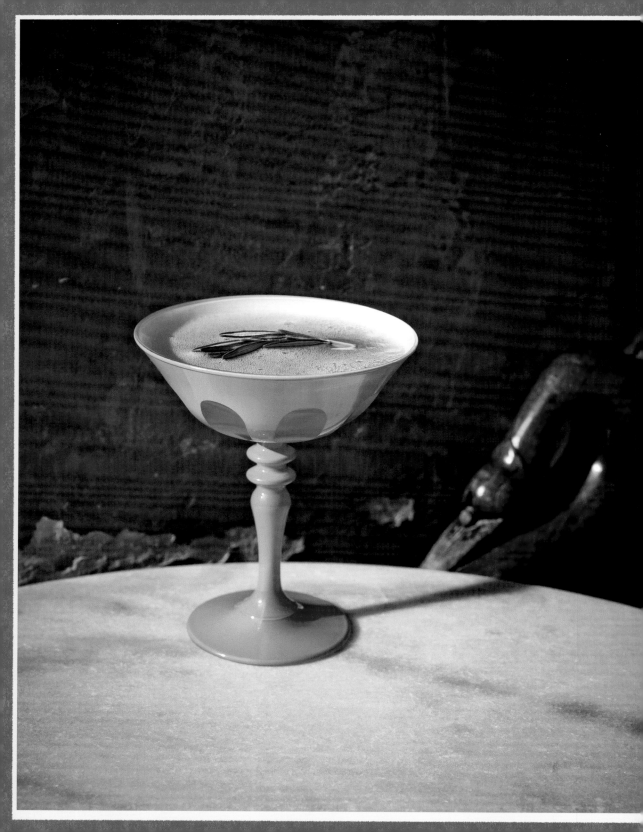

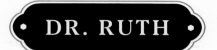

# · DR. RUTH ·

*The Dr. Ruth is a seasonally versatile cocktail. The rosemary is reminiscent of Thanksgiving and Christmas dishes, and the strawberry of summer fields. Combine Rosemary-Infused Vodka with Strawberry Purée, top with a bit of Champagne, and you have one of the most successful cocktails on our menu.*

### FORMULA

2 ounces Rosemary-Infused Vodka
*(page 234)*

1 ounce Strawberry Purée *(page 231)*

1 ounce Sour Mix *(page 227)*

Champagne

Garnish rosemary sprig

### TOOLS

Jigger

Shaker

Hawthorne strainer

Coupe glass

### EXECUTION

**Combine all of the measured ingredients in a shaker with ice. Shake vigorously and strain into a coupe glass. Top with Champagne and garnish with a rosemary sprig.**

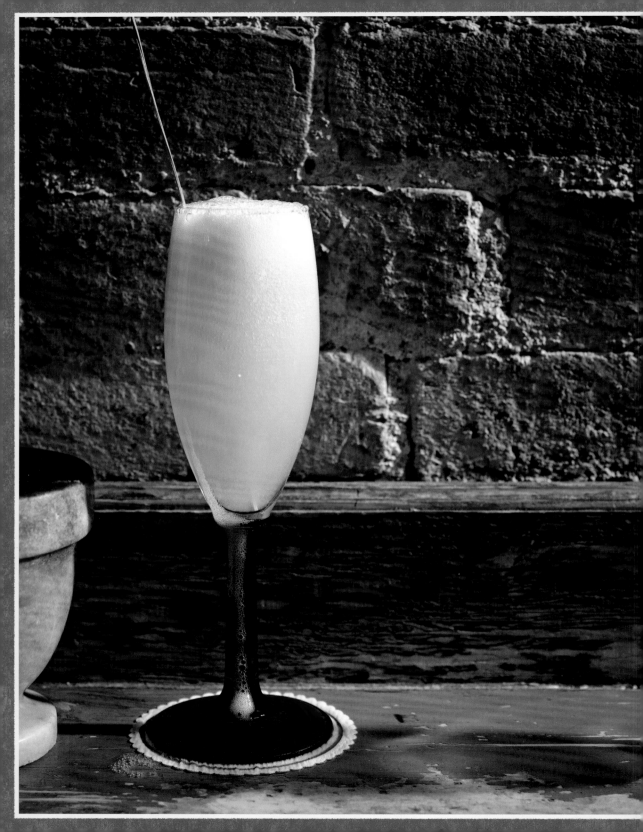

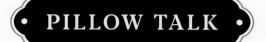

# PILLOW TALK

*The bison grass garnish always generates some buzz. The seed for this drink was planted when one of our doormen suggested creating a white drink and naming it Pillow Talk. In the end, the drink wasn't white, but we kept the fun name. Usually the process of creating a cocktail is iterative, with several different versions and much tweaking to achieve perfection. However, this drink was an anomaly of sorts: it was the fastest drink that we designed and loved right away. The sweet and intriguing flavor of the bison grass vodka makes it shine, and the bison grass garnish has a delicate and subtle aroma.*

### FORMULA

2 ounces bison grass vodka

1½ ounces Honeydew Purée
*(page 230)*

½ ounce Sour Mix *(page 227)*

Champagne

Garnish bison grass

### TOOLS

Jigger

Shaker

Hawthorne strainer

Flute glass

### EXECUTION

**Add all of the measured ingredients to a shaker with ice. Shake vigorously and strain into a flute glass. Top with Champagne and garnish with a piece of bison grass.**

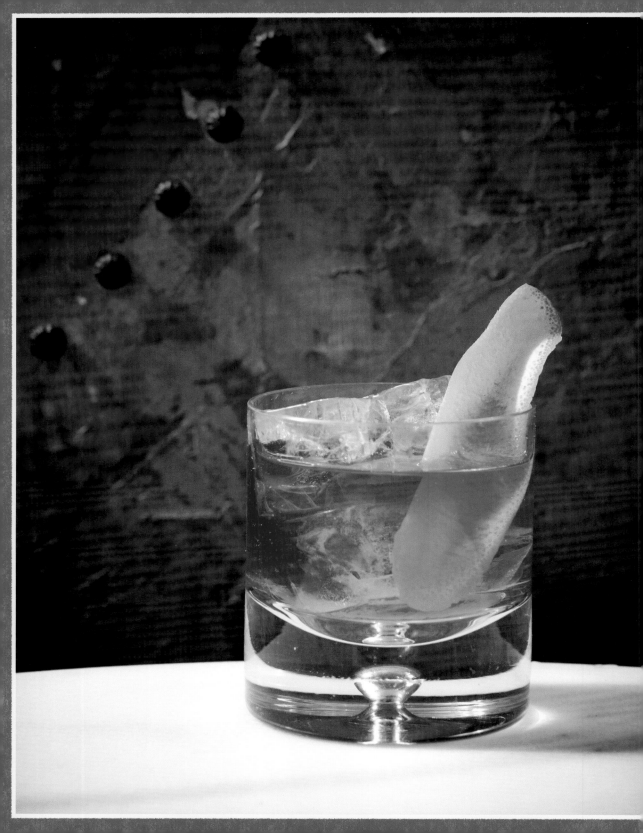

# • VANILLA-SAFFRON OLD-FASHIONED

We wanted to pay homage to the old-fashioned—one of the classic, original cocktails—
so we designed one with sultry ingredients. Old-fashioned cocktails always use
bourbon, although some people have started to experiment with rye now that the latter
has gained in popularity, recovering from its post-Prohibition slump. This is one of the
only cocktails in this chapter that does not require shaking. Since it is a spirit-forward
drink, it employs stirring instead.

## FORMULA

Orange peel

Dollop agave nectar

Dash Angostura bitters

3 ounces Vanilla and Saffron–Infused
Bourbon *(page 234)*

## TOOLS

Citrus peeler

Rocks glass

Muddler

Jigger

Bar spoon

## EXECUTION

Rub the orange peel along the rim of a rocks glass. Drop the orange zest into the
glass and add the agave and bitters. Coat the inside of the glass using a muddler.
Add the bourbon and 2 ice cubes. Stir for approximately 50 rotations until the
liquid is thoroughly chilled. Add 2 fresh ice cubes on top and serve.

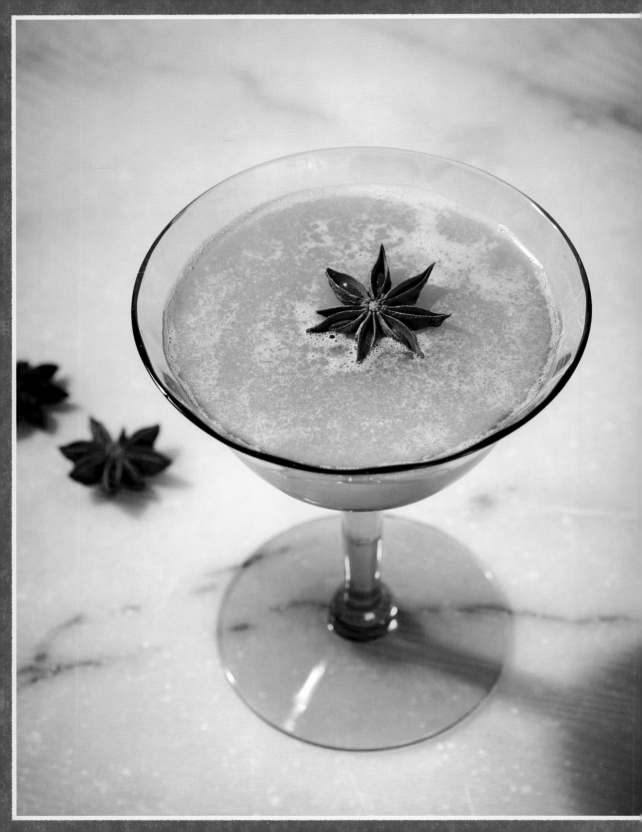

# • STUNT DOUBLE •

*Bourbon and peach are a classic southern combination, and we deepen the complexity of the flavors by smoking white peaches and adding a dash of absinthe.*

### FORMULA

2 ounces bourbon

1 ounce Hickory-Smoked
White Peach Purée *(page 235)*

1 ounce Sour Mix *(page 227)*

Dash absinthe

Garnish star anise

### TOOLS

Jigger

Shaker

Hawthorne strainer

Tea strainer

Coupe glass

### EXECUTION

**Add all measured ingredients to a shaker with ice. Shake vigorously and double strain into a coupe glass. Garnish with star anise.**

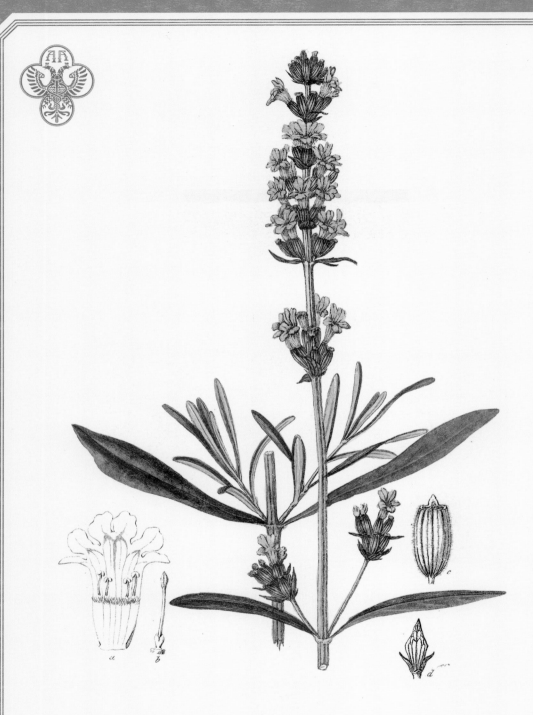

*Lavandula Spica.*

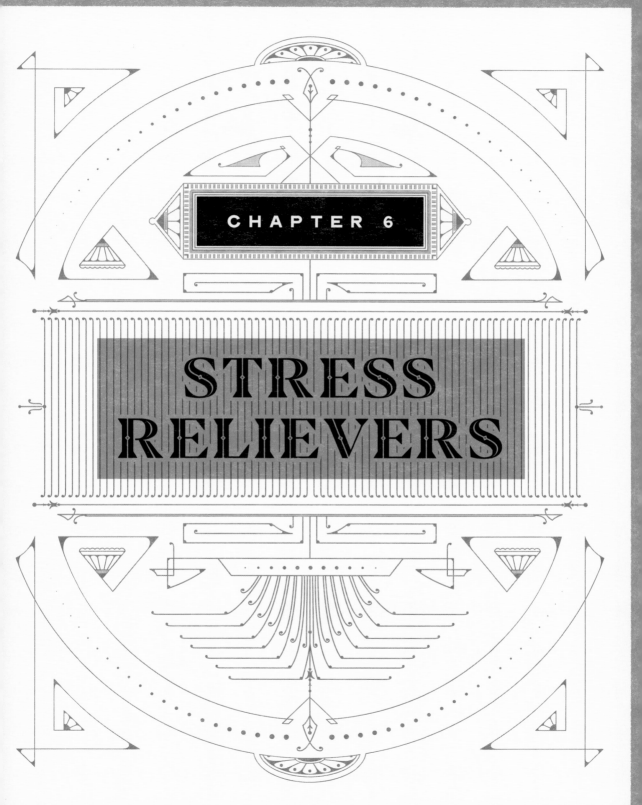

CHAPTER 6

# STRESS RELIEVERS

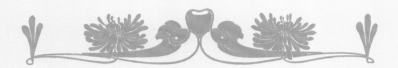

**P**LANTS ARE OUR FRIENDS. IN A 2018 *TIME* ARTICLE, plants are described as "indispensable" to human life. Through photosynthesis, they produce life-giving oxygen and remove harmful toxins from the air we breathe. They also combat stress and anxiety. Stress is a silent killer. Numerous studies demonstrate a clear link between high stress and health issues.

We should take note: many ancient cultures used calming teas and other herb preparations to keep their stress at bay.

## Traits of Ingredients in This Chapter

Perhaps the most well-known stress-relieving botanical is lavender. In clinical trials, participants' cortisol, a stress hormone, was shown to be greatly reduced within five minutes of smelling fresh lavender. Likewise, essential oils from lavender, lemongrass, and other stress-relieving plants are widely produced for use in aromatherapy treatments for their calming and relaxing properties.

One of the most ancient medicinal herbs known to mankind, and another well-known stress-relieving plant, is chamomile. In addition to scent, the stress-relieving properties of chamomile are often experienced through its most

popular form—herbal tea—and humans consume more than one million cups per day. Hibiscus, another popular tea-administered, stress-relieving plant, helps cardiovascular circulation by widening arteries, which increases blood flow.

## Spirit Notes

Any alcohol can be a stress reliever, of course. Some of our stress-relieving drinks naturally gravitate toward rum, which makes sense given rum's Caribbean roots (the region's crystal-clear turquoise waters and lush forests are big draws for vacationers). Rum is also a sugarcane-based spirit, and we all know that sugar is a tantalizing stress reliever.

In this section of our menu, we showcase well-known and unique stress-relieving ingredients in a balanced presentation designed to calm the mind and body.

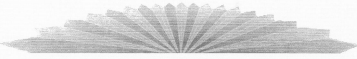

FEATURED STRESS-RELIEVING BOTANICALS

# CARDAMOM

# CHAMOMILE

# HIBISCUS

# LAVENDER

# LEMONGRASS

*Alcohol prompts the release of our brain's happy chemicals—endorphins—*
*which produce feelings of pleasure.*

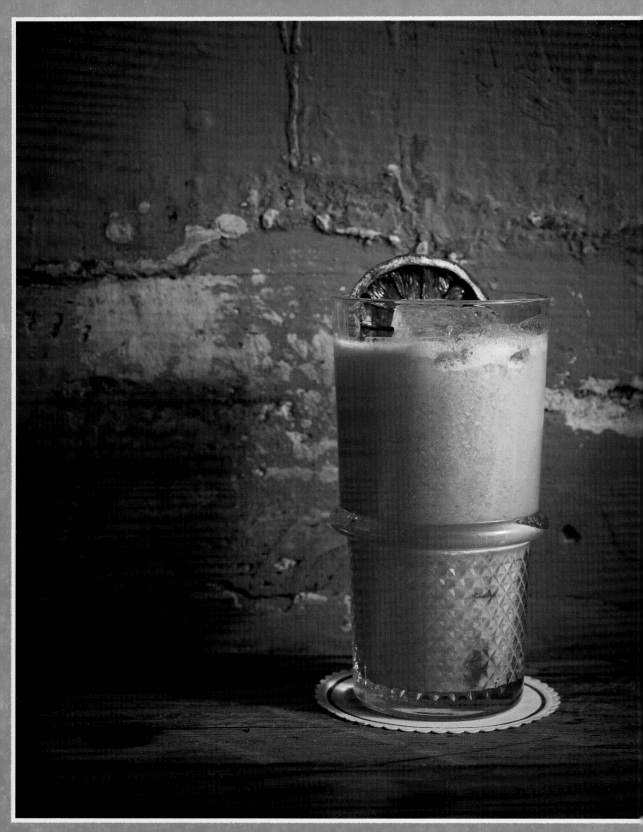

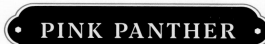

# · PINK PANTHER ·

*Palo santo has a distinctive, earthy aroma. After smoking fruits and other botanicals, we decided to experiment with smoking liquids to see if they would taste like they smelled. The verdict? They did indeed. Palo santo gives the rum a fantastic scent. This is one of our sweeter creations, with echoes of a piña colada, but with guava and blood orange replacing the pineapple. With its lovely pink hue and accessible ingredients, it attracts the sly and sexy.*

### FORMULA

2 ounces Palo Santo–Smoked Rum
*(page 235)*

1 ounce Guava–Blood Orange Purée
*(page 230)*

¾ ounce sweetened coconut milk

¾ ounce Sour Mix *(page 227)*

Garnish dehydrated blood
orange wheel

### TOOLS

Jigger

Shaker

Hawthorne strainer

Collins glass

### EXECUTION

Add all measured ingredients to a shaker with ice. Shake vigorously and strain into a Collins glass with fresh ice. Garnish with a dehydrated blood orange wheel.

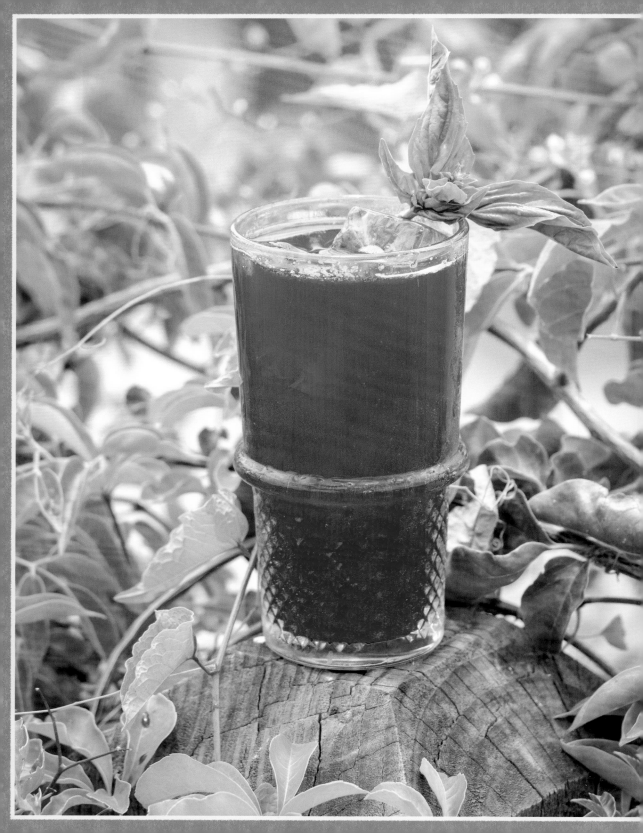

# • MIRACLE OF MAZUNTE •

*The Oaxacan beach town of Mazunte perfectly embodies this cocktail's soul of deep Mexican flavors and Caribbean tropical bite. Calling all of its fresh and smoky qualities from the earth, notes of beet, basil, and mezcal are uplifted by sour and spice, all topped off with club soda to refresh in any climate.*

## FORMULA

2 basil leaves

2 ounces Basil-Infused Mezcal
*(page 232)*

1 ounce beet juice

¾ ounce lime juice

½ ounce Simple Syrup *(page 226)*

3 dashes Habanero Tincture
*(page 228)*

1½ cc APO Cerebral Bitters
*(recommended)*

Top with club soda

Garnish basil leaf

## TOOLS

Shaker

Jigger

Lemon squeezer

Hawthorne strainer

Collins glass

## EXECUTION

**Tear the basil leaves and place in a shaker. Add the measured ingredients to the shaker with ice. Shake vigorously. Add club soda and then strain ingredients into a Collins glass over fresh ice. Garnish with a whole basil leaf.**

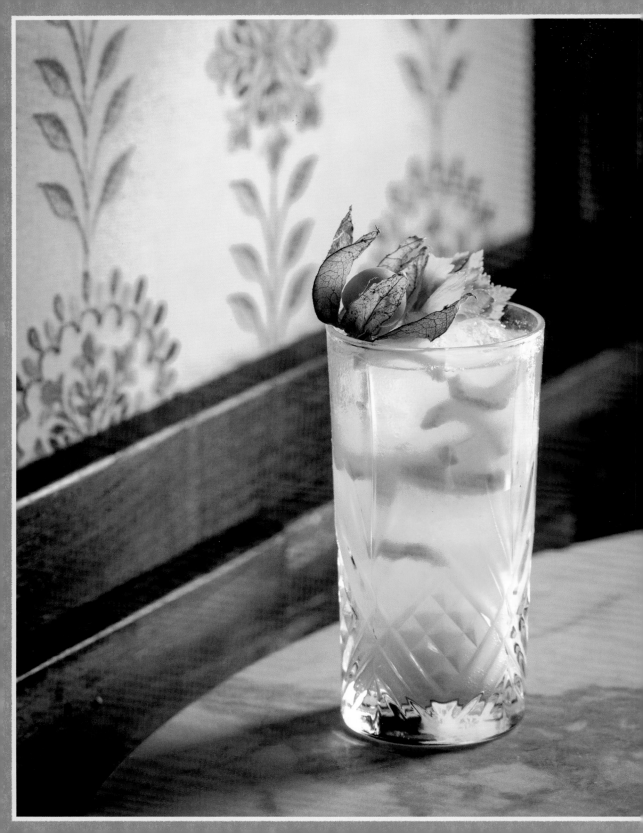

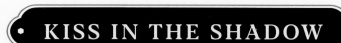

# · KISS IN THE SHADOW ·

CREATED EXCLUSIVELY FOR THIS BOOK

*Each fresh ingredient gets a bright moment to reveal its wonderfully unique and delicious taste before giving way to the next piece in this balanced dance of the palate. Flavor awaits at every turn, as the notes revolve in seductive order. All patiently awaiting their moment to strike the senses.*

## FORMULA

2 gooseberries
2 stalks celery
2 ounces rum
¼ ounce aquavit
½ ounce Cantaloupe Purée *(page 229)*
1 ounce royal milk tea *(see note)*
½ ounce lime juice
½ ounce Simple Syrup *(page 226)*
Pinch sea salt
Top with club soda
Garnish gooseberry, sliced celery

## TOOLS

Muddler
Shaker
Jigger
Lemon squeezer
Hawthorne strainer
Collins glass

NOTE: Royal milk tea is readily available for purchase online.

## EXECUTION

**Muddle the gooseberries and celery in a shaker. Add the remaining measured ingredients and salt to the shaker with ice and shake vigorously. Pour club soda into the shaker and strain into a Collins glass with fresh ice. Add the garnishes.**

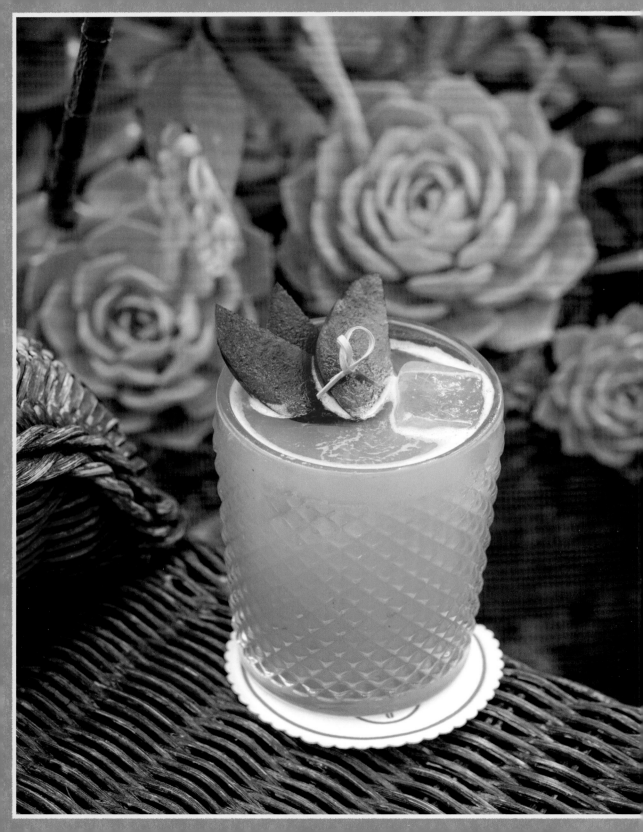

# • RED-HANDED HOWLER •

*In ancient Mayan culture, the howler monkey was believed to be the divine patron of artisans. At Apotheke we offer up this tart, fresh blend of red plum, lime, and cardamom balanced with the woody strength of Scotch to artisans and monkeys alike.*

## FORMULA

1¾ ounces Scotch

¼ ounce pox *(see note)*

¼ ounce Rosolio di Bergamotto
*(see note)*

1 ounce Plum-Cardamom Purée
*(page 231)*

½ ounce lime juice

½ ounce Simple Syrup *(page 226)*

1 cc APO Cerebral Bitters
*(recommended)*

Garnish plum slices

## TOOLS

Jigger

Lemon squeezer

Shaker

Hawthorne strainer

Rocks glass

## EXECUTION

**Add all measured ingredients to a shaker with ice. Shake vigorously. Strain into a rocks glass with fresh ice. Garnish with a fan of plum slices.**

NOTE: Pox is a Mexican corn-based spirit, sometimes with sugarcane and/or wheat added, rooted in centuries-old Mayan rituals and medicinal uses. Rosolio di Bergamotto is a light, sweet Italian aperitif flavored with citrus, rose, and aromatic herbs.

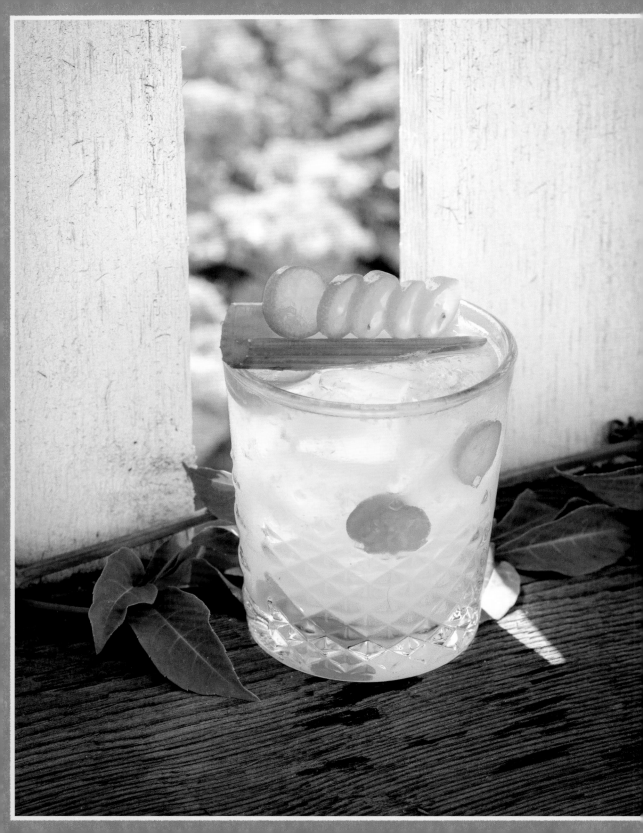

# SUNBURNED HAND OF THE MAN

CREATED BY WALTON GOGGINS AND NICOLAS O'CONNOR

*Starting with the sturdy botanical notes of gin, this libation weaves its tale up from a savory ground to the exotic, fruity heights of the passion fruit vine. Tart and sweet, but also delicate and smooth, this cocktail will have you basking in the sunshine.*

## FORMULA

2 stalks celery

2 kumquats

Pinch sea salt

2 ounces Buddha's Hand–Infused Gin
*(page 232)*

¼ ounce Rosolio di Bergamotto *(see note)*

½ ounce Passion Fruit Purée *(page 230)*

½ ounce lime juice

¼ ounce Simple Syrup *(page 226)*

Garnish kumquat and celery stalk

## TOOLS

Muddler

Shaker

Jigger

Lemon squeezer

Hawthorne strainer

Rocks glass

## EXECUTION

**Muddle the celery and kumquats in a shaker. Add a pinch of sea salt.**
**Add all measured ingredients to the shaker with ice. Shake vigorously.**
**Strain ingredients into a rocks glass with fresh ice. Add the garnish.**

NOTE: Rosolio di Bergamotto is a light, sweet Italian aperitif flavored with citrus, rose, and aromatic herbs.

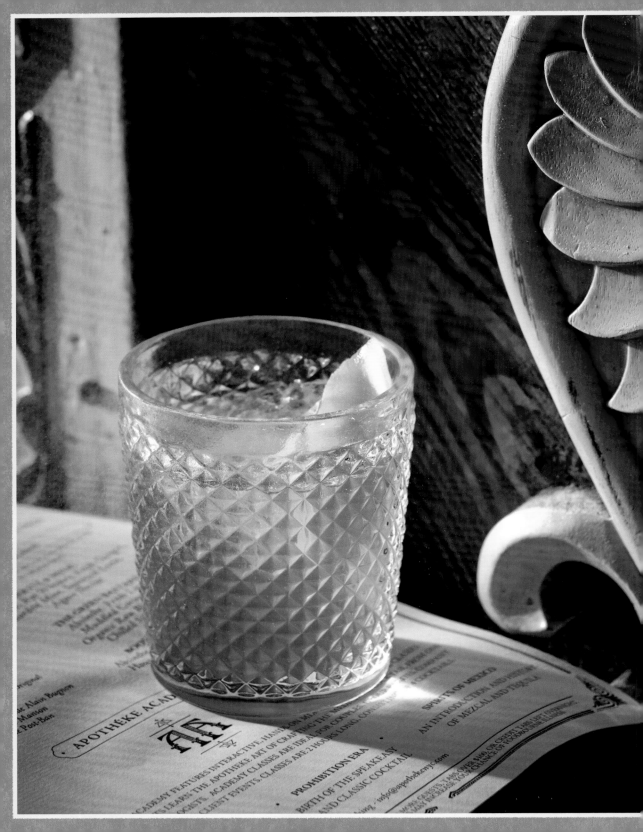

# • CATCHER IN THE RYE •

*The Catcher in the Rye is one of our bestsellers. Although the book was once banned, the stirred spirits in this blend shall not be forgotten. The amaro softens the rye, creating a base that allows the chamomile cordial and peated Scotch to perfectly balance it all.*

<table>
<tr><td>

**FORMULA**

2 ounces rye

½ ounce Amaro Nonino

½ ounce Honey-Chamomile Cordial
*(page 227)*

Peated Scotch *(mist)*

Garnish lemon peel

</td><td>

**TOOLS**

Jigger

Mixing glass

Bar spoon

Julep strainer

Rocks glass

Atomizer

Citrus peeler

</td></tr>
</table>

**EXECUTION**

**Add the measured ingredients to a mixing glass with ice. Stir approximately 50 rotations, until the liquid is thoroughly chilled; strain into a rocks glass with fresh ice. Fill the atomizer with peated Scotch and mist over the glass. Garnish with the lemon peel.**

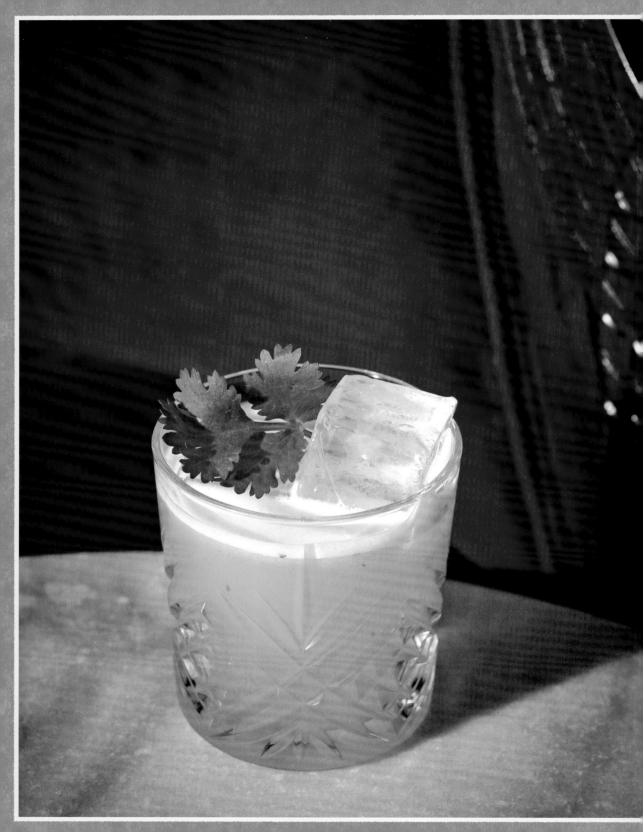

# • SITTING BUDDHA •

*This is one of the most enduring drinks on our menu. The lemongrass is subtle, delicate, and calming, and the strokes of pineapple and cilantro create the bold and refreshing allure of our most popular cocktail.*

## FORMULA

2 ounces Lemongrass-Infused Vodka *(page 233)*
1 ounce Pineapple Purée *(page 231)*
½ ounce Ginger Mix *(page 226)*
1 ounce Sour Mix *(page 227)*
3 sprigs cilantro
Garnish cilantro sprig

## TOOLS

Jigger
Shaker
Hawthorne strainer
Rocks glass

## EXECUTION

Add all measured ingredients and the three sprigs of cilantro to a shaker with ice. Shake vigorously and strain into a rocks glass with fresh ice. Garnish with a sprig of cilantro.

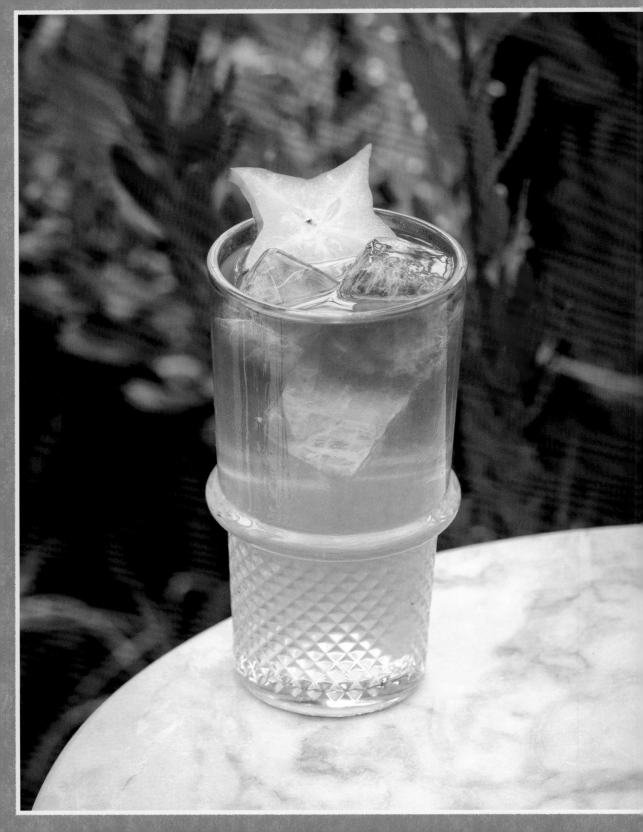

# • COSMONAUT •

*The Cosmonaut is our attempt to add depth and distinction to the Moscow mule and send the palate to outer space. The added floral and tart notes launch this libation into uncharted flavor galaxies. Using crisp star fruit with bright hibiscus enriches the earthy ginger spice, all of which is orbited with heavenly scented Lavender-Infused Vodka.*

## FORMULA

2 slices star fruit

2 ounces Lavender-Infused Vodka
*(page 233)*

¾ ounce Ginger Water *(page 226)*

¾ ounce lime juice

¾ ounce Simple Syrup *(page 226)*

Top with ginger beer

Float ¼ ounce Hibiscus Tincture
*(page 228)*

Garnish star fruit

## TOOLS

Muddler

Shaker

Jigger

Lemon squeezer

Hawthorne strainer

Collins glass

Bar spoon

## EXECUTION

**Muddle the star fruit in a shaker. Add the vodka, Ginger Water, lime juice, and Simple Syrup to the shaker with ice. Shake vigorously. Add the ginger beer to the shaker. Strain the contents into a Collins glass with fresh ice. Add a Hibiscus Tincture float (see tip) and garnish with a piece of star fruit.**

HOW TO EXECUTE A FLOAT: Slowly pour the liquid over the back of a bar spoon, holding the spoon just above the liquid you are topping.

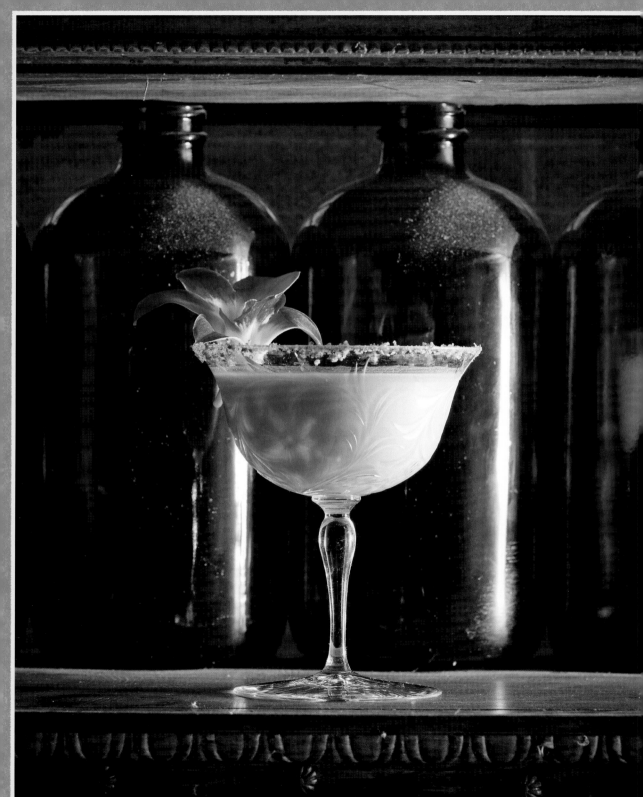

# • SUNDARA SOUR •

*Channel the flavors and aromas of India with this creation. The Mango Lassi has fruit and goat-milk yogurt, which offers fantastic body since it is dry and sour.*

## FORMULA

2 ounces Sundara-Infused Gin
*(page 234)*

2¾ ounces Mango Lassi Purée
*(page 230)*

½ ounce Sour Mix *(page 227)*

Lime wedge

Curry Salt *(page 235)*

Garnish purple orchid

## TOOLS

Jigger

Shaker

Coupe glass

Hawthorne strainer

## EXECUTION

Add the gin, Mango Lassi, and Sour Mix to a shaker with ice and shake.
Use a lime wedge to coat half the circumference of the rim of a coupe glass
and then dip it into the curry salt. Strain the contents of the shaker into the
coupe glass. Garnish with the orchid.

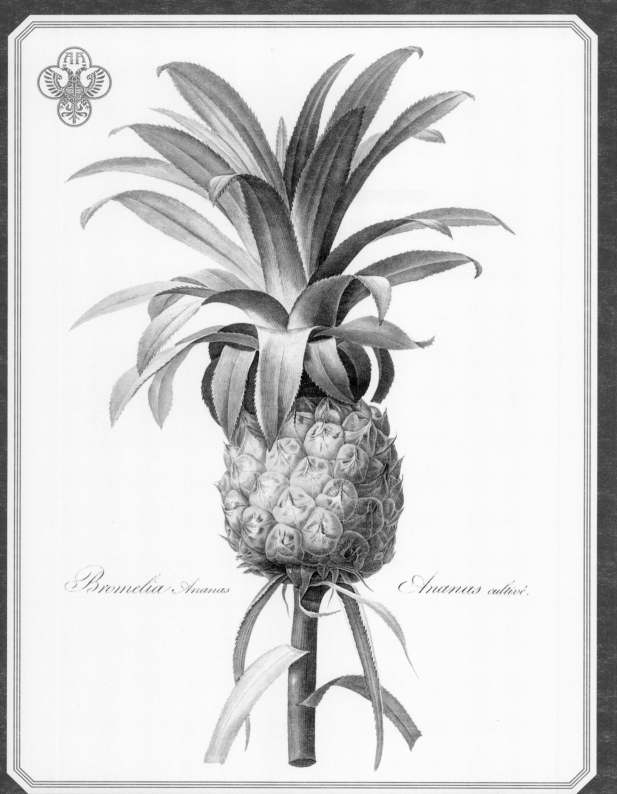

*Bromelia Ananas*          *Ananas cultivé.*

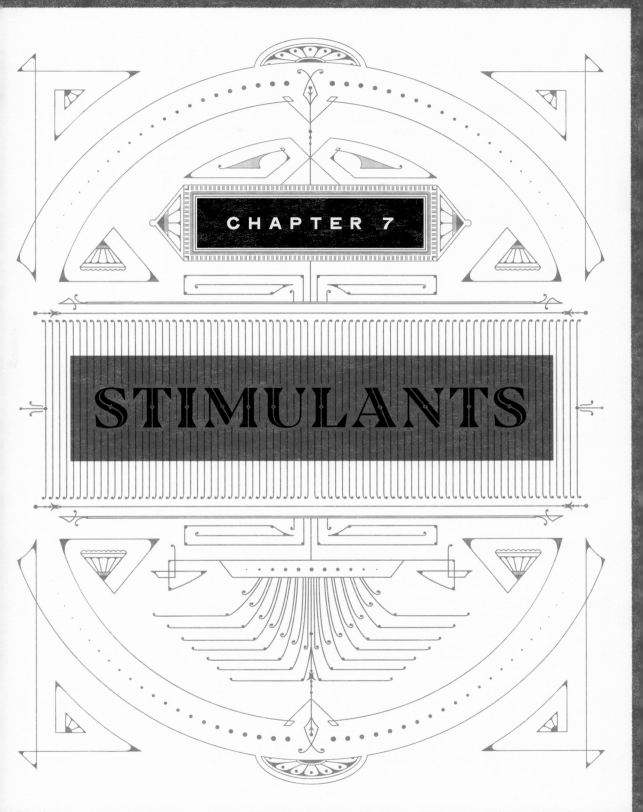

CHAPTER 7

STIMULANTS

*The divine drink, which builds up resistance and fights fatigue. A cup of this precious drink [cocoa] permits man to walk for a whole day without food.*

—Aztec emperor Montezuma II
(reign: 1502–1520)

**H**UMANS ACROSS TIME AND GEOGRAPHY HAVE AT LEAST this in common: they seek out stimulants and ways to boost their alertness and stamina. Indigenous tribes in the Americas discovered coca (eventually to inspire Coca-Cola and cocaine), which made its way into American pharmacies in the nineteenth century before being banned.

When we think of stimulants, coffee comes to mind. Caffeine increases the release of catecholamines (such as adrenaline) via the sympathetic nervous system, which, among other things, can make your heart beat faster, sending more blood to your muscles and telling your liver to release sugar into the bloodstream for energy. Caffeine, one of humankind's favorite stimulants, is a fascinating chemical. It is technically a poison produced by the plant; you could die if you drank fifty cups of coffee in one sitting.

## Traits of Ingredients in This Chapter

Pineapple has high levels of vitamin $B_6$, which helps stabilize the body's blood sugar, along with manganese and thiamine, which aid in energy production.

Watermelon is a great source of B vitamins and fiber, as well as water, which is key to maintaining one's energy. Watermelon helps rehydrate your body. Watermelons also contain an amino acid called citrulline, which gets converted into arginine when absorbed by the body and helps improve blood flow, providing more energy.

Cantaloupe is a great source of B vitamins and fiber, as well as water, which is key to pretty much everything, including maintaining your energy. Eating melon can help rehydrate your body.

Cucumber is low in calories but contains many important vitamins and minerals and has a high water content. Eating cucumbers may lead to many potential health benefits, including weight loss, balanced hydration, digestive regularity, and lower blood sugar levels.

## Spirit Notes

Mezcal and tequila are key spirits for our stimulating drinks. The agave they contain is a natural stimulant.

In this section, we explore how stimulation can be paired with alcohol to invigorate the body and mind.

### FEATURED STIMULANT BOTANICALS

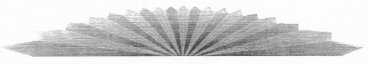

# COFFEE

# PINEAPPLE

# WATERMELON

# CANTALOUPE

# CUCUMBER

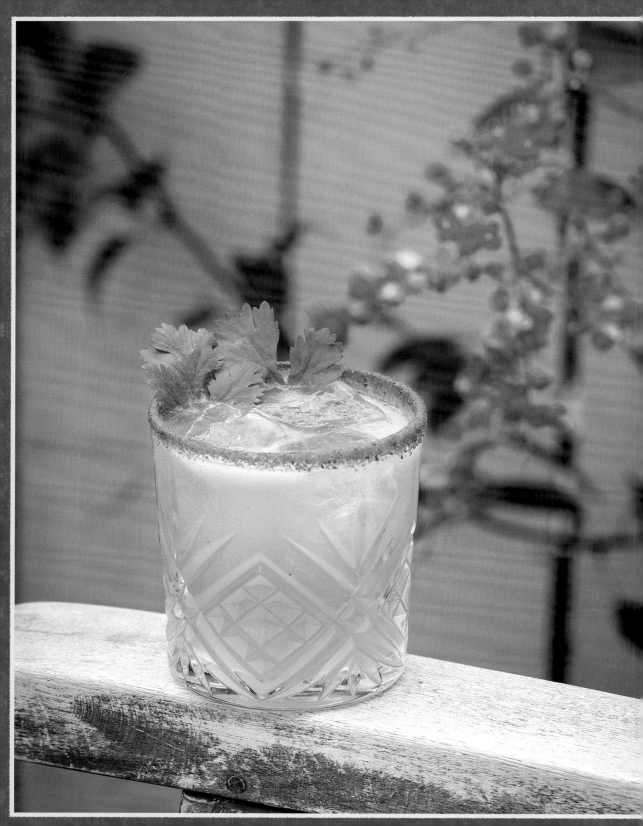

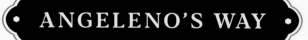

# • ANGELENO'S WAY •

*This is a cool, fresh, and laid-back Los Angeles breeze of fruit and botanicals with a savory, popping street spice from our neighbors down south. It's an homage to the spicy fruit blends sold by street vendors throughout the City of Angels. Truly the Angeleno's way.*

### FORMULA

4 to 6 sprigs cilantro

2 ounces Cilantro-Infused Tequila
*(page 232)*

1 ounce watermelon juice

¾ ounce lime juice

½ ounce Simple Syrup *(page 226)*

2 dashes Habanero Tincture *(page 228)*

1 dash Bilberry Tincture *(page 228)*

1½ cc APO Rejuvenation Bitters
*(recommended)*

Wedge blood orange or other citrus

Rim Old Bay Seasoning

Garnish cilantro

### TOOLS

Shaker

Jigger

Lemon squeezer

Rocks glass

Hawthorne strainer

Tea strainer

### EXECUTION

Tear and place the cilantro leaves into a shaker. Add the remaining measured ingredients to the shaker with ice. Shake vigorously. Rub the rim of a rocks glass with a wedge of blood orange and evenly rim the glass with Old Bay Seasoning. Double strain the ingredients over fresh ice into the rimmed rocks glass. Add garnish.

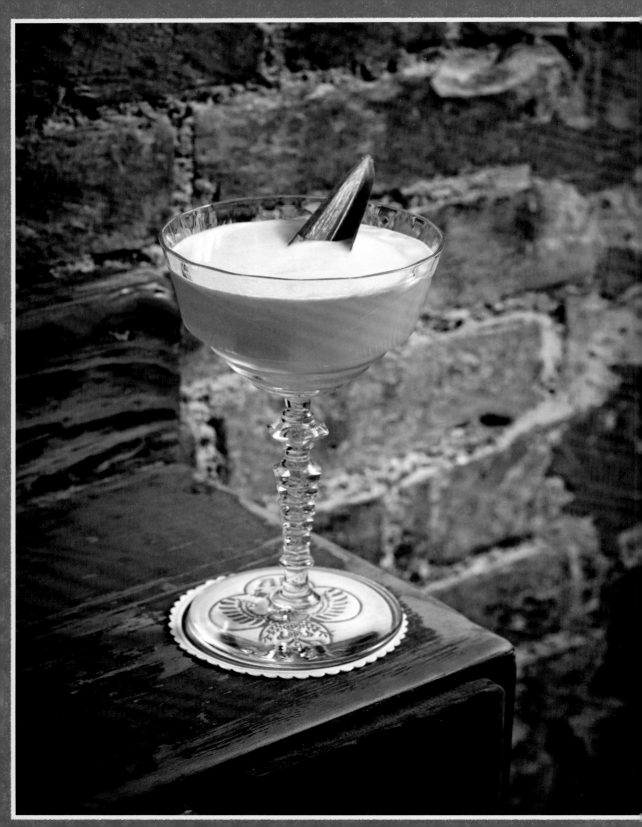

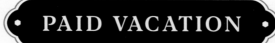

# PAID VACATION

*This beauty started as an experiment to see if we could use a barbecue smoker for fresh fruit. As it turns out, we could. Hickory-smoked pineapple is one aspect of a small cocktail with a big flavor. Paired with equal parts mezcal and tequila, as well as our house-made bitters, this one covers all aspects of the flavor profile. Muddled cucumber gives it a brightness, and the smoky pineapple and mezcal are reminiscent of a cookout in Cancun. Wrap that up with a spicy kick at the end, and you're on a paid vacation.*

## FORMULA

3 cucumber wheels, ¼ inch thick

1 ounce blanco tequila

1 ounce mezcal

1 ounce Hickory-Smoked Pineapple Purée *(page 235)*

1 ounce Sour Mix *(page 227)*

½ ounce Habanero Tincture *(page 228)*

Garnish pineapple leaf

## TOOLS

Muddler

Shaker

Jigger

Hawthorne strainer

Tea strainer

Coupe glass

## EXECUTION

**Muddle the cucumber wheels in a shaker. Add all of the measured ingredients to the shaker with ice. Shake vigorously. Double strain into a coupe glass. Garnish with a pineapple leaf.**

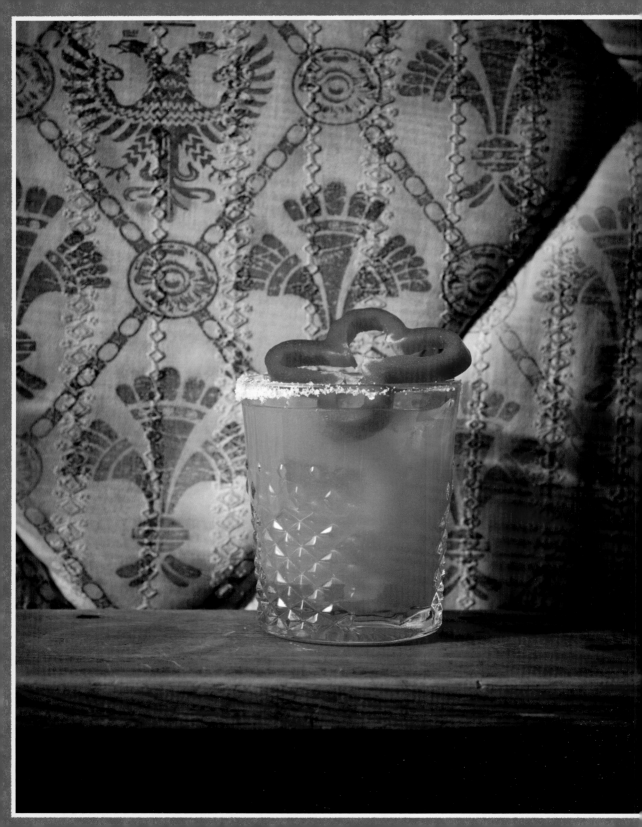

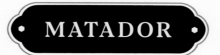

# · MATADOR ·

*This cocktail adds the zesty pop of red bell pepper and the subtle, sweet flavor of cantaloupe to a classic margarita.*

## FORMULA

2 red bell pepper rings

2 ounces reposado tequila

1½ ounces Cantaloupe Purée
*(page 229)*

1 ounce Sour Mix *(page 227)*

½ ounce Habanero Tincture
*(page 228)*

Orange slice

Rim Sambuca and Anise Sea Salt
*(page 236)*

Garnish red bell pepper and cracked
black pepper

## TOOLS

Muddler

Shaker

Jigger

Rocks glass

Hawthorne strainer

Tea strainer

## EXECUTION

Muddle the red pepper rings in a shaker. Add the measured ingredients to the shaker with ice and shake vigorously. Rub the rim of a rocks glass with an orange slice and rim the glass with Sambuca and Anise Sea Salt. Double strain into the glass. Garnish with a red pepper ring and cracked black pepper.

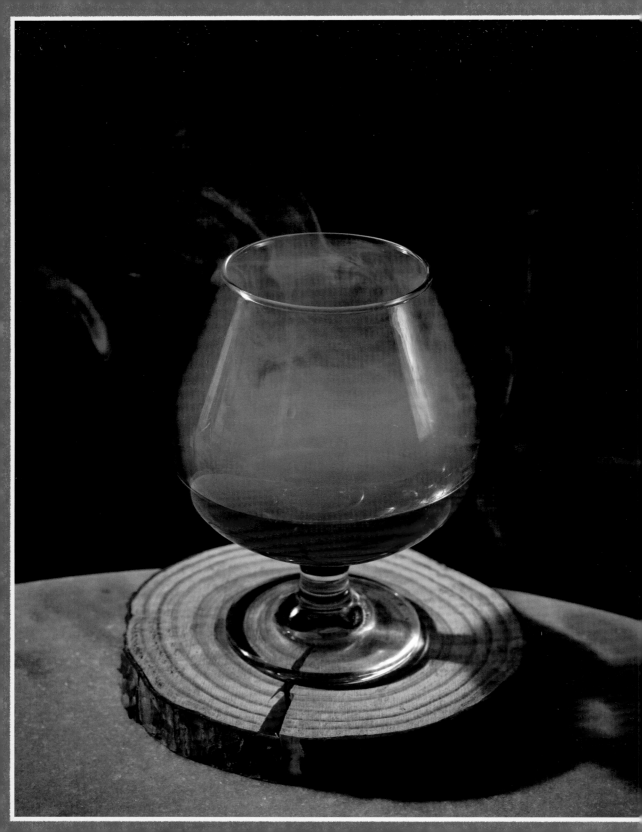

# • DEAD POET •

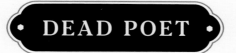

*Smoke was in spirit. The unforgettable Dead Poet is one of our most photographed and videoed creations. It was carefully designed to make you feel like you're happily stranded at a winter cabin, snuggled up next to a fire. The cozy fragrance of the smoking cloves and spectacle of presenting the drink—burning the cloves under a brandy snifter so the smell permeates the glass—always makes guests say, "Give me that fiery, smoking one!"*

## FORMULA

1½ ounces Espresso, Black Walnut
Husk, and Allspice–Infused Bourbon
*(page 233)*

1½ ounces rye

Dash agave nectar

Cloves

## TOOLS

Jigger

Mixing glass

Bar spoon

Oakwood disk *(see note)*

Kitchen torch

Snifter glass

Julep strainer

## EXECUTION

**Combine the bourbon, rye, and nectar in a mixing glass with ice. Stir approximately 50 rotations until the liquid is thoroughly chilled. Lay a pinch of cloves on the oak disk and ignite until they smoke. Cover the cloves with a snifter until the inside of the glass is full of smoke. Remove the glass, turning it right-side up, and strain the contents of the mixing glass into it.**

NOTE: Oakwood disks (see photograph on opposite page) can be sourced online.

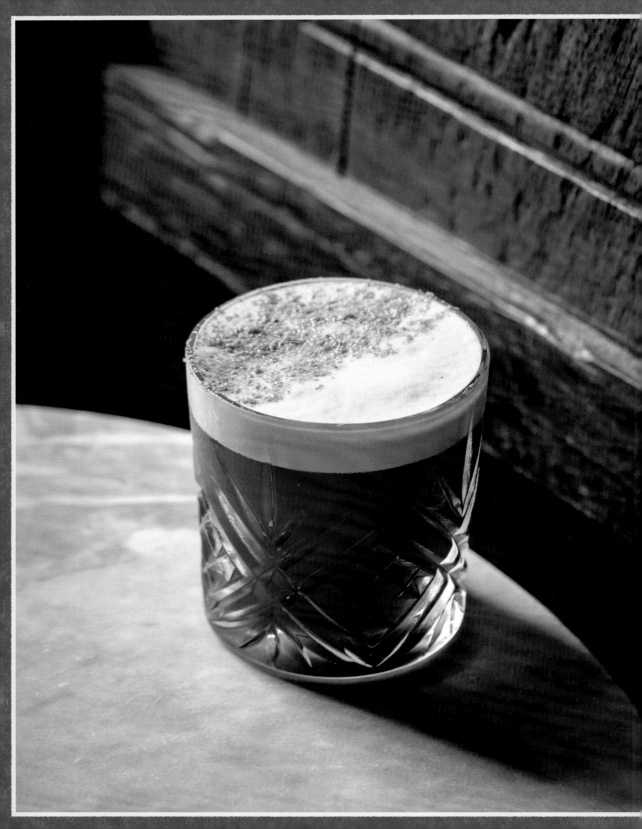

# • COFFEE AND CIGARETTES •

*A cup of coffee and a cigarette. That legendary pair are ever entwined in an astringent dance of feel and flavor. To capture that essence, we infuse our base spirit with coffee, catching the beginning of the palate. This blends into the tobacco bitters, which linger till the end. To balance this journey, we uplift with black cherry and lime while stabilizing the texture with rum and egg whites.*

## FORMULA

1½ ounces Coffee-Infused Scotch
*(page 232)*

½ ounce molasses-based rum

¾ ounce black cherry juice

¾ ounce egg whites

½ ounce lime juice

½ ounce Simple Syrup *(page 226)*

2 dashes Bitter Queens Tobacco
Bitters

Garnish Ground Pistachios Mix
*(page 235)*

## TOOLS

Jigger

Shaker

Hawthorne strainer

Tea strainer

Rocks glass

## EXECUTION

**Add all of the measured ingredients to a shaker with ice. Shake vigorously.
Double strain the contents of the shaker into a rocks glass with fresh ice.
Sprinkle the pistachio mix over the top.**

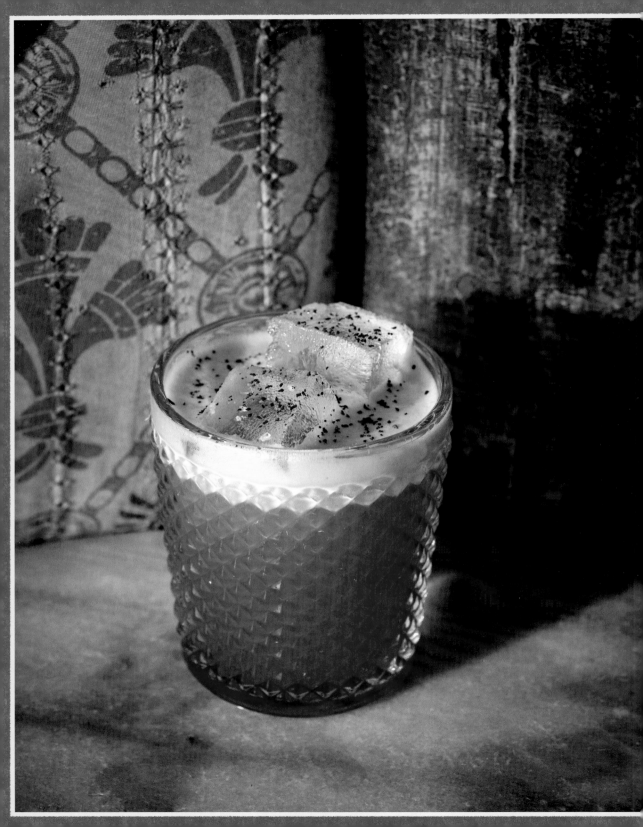

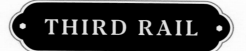

# · THIRD RAIL ·

*An NYC take on a dark and stormy with a jolt of electricity. Coffee and booze, the lifeblood*
*of New Yorkers, are generously blended together to give you your wants and needs.*

## FORMULA

2 ounces black rum

1 ounce chilled fresh-brewed coffee

1 ounce Ginger Mix *(page 226)*

1 ounce Sour Mix *(page 227)*

Garnish coffee grounds

## TOOLS

Jigger

Shaker

Hawthorne strainer

Rocks glass

## EXECUTION

**Add all of the measured ingredients to a shaker with ice. Shake vigorously and**
**strain into a rocks glass with fresh ice. Garnish with fresh coffee grounds.**

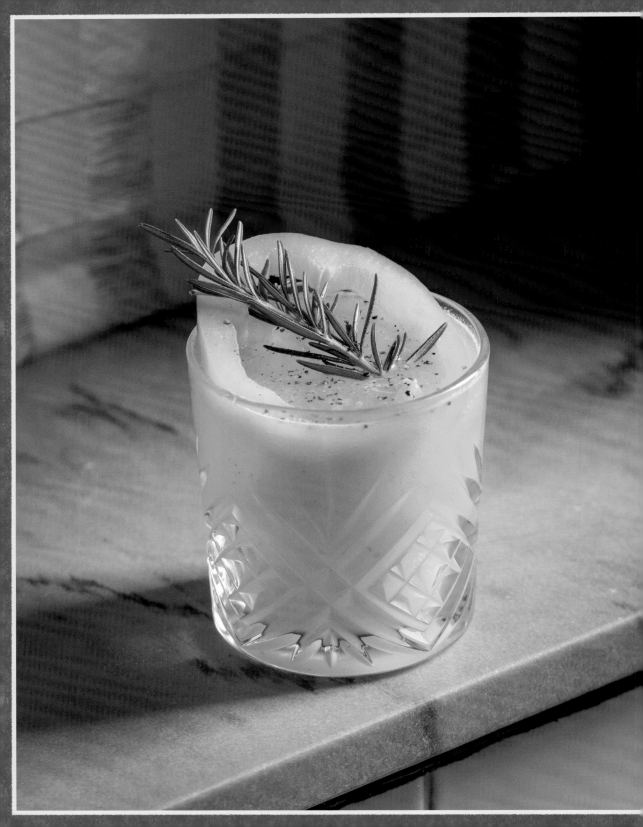

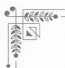
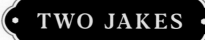

# • TWO JAKES •

*For over a century, adventurers have sought the riches held within the gold mine of the Lost Dutchman, named for two inspirational seekers who discovered this cache of gold. We, too, sought those riches and found earthy and sweet golden beets, tangy and juicy nectarines, and crisp yellow bell peppers. Two Jakes perfectly blends these flavors and the yearning for gold that this pair of adventurers surely felt.*

## FORMULA

2 rings yellow bell pepper

2 ounces tequila

1½ ounces Nectarine–Golden Beet Purée *(page 230)*

¾ ounce lime juice

¾ ounce Simple Syrup *(page 226)*

2 dashes Habanero Tincture *(page 228)*

Cracked black pepper

Garnish rosemary sprig and yellow bell pepper

## TOOLS

Muddler

Shaker

Jigger

Hawthorne strainer

Rocks glass

## EXECUTION

**Muddle the yellow bell pepper in a shaker. Add all of the measured ingredients to the shaker with ice. Shake vigorously. Strain the contents into a rocks glass with fresh ice. Crack the pepper over the top. Garnish with a rosemary sprig and yellow bell pepper ring.**

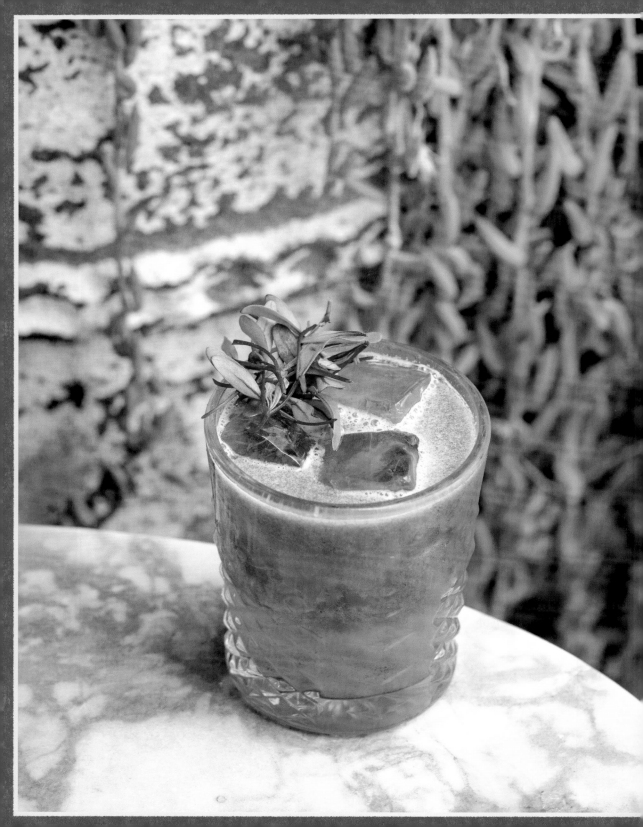

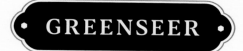

# • GREENSEER •

*Look to the future. The right amount of the superfood spirulina accompanied with bright produce and the bold power of agave-based spirits creates a harmonious experience. It looks like a smoothie with its deep, lustrous color, but actually has a light viscosity allowing all of the ingredients to flow.*

### FORMULA

1 ounce tequila

1 ounce mezcal

1 ounce Honeydew-Spirulina Purée
*(page 230)*

½ ounce lime juice

½ ounce Simple Syrup *(page 226)*

2 dashes Habanero Tincture
*(page 228)*

Garnish 6 to 8 micro bull's
blood beet greens

### TOOLS

Jigger

Lemon squeezer

Shaker

Hawthorne strainer

Rocks glass

### EXECUTION

**Add all of the measured ingredients to a shaker with ice. Shake vigorously. Strain the ingredients into a rocks glass with fresh ice. Garnish with micro bull's blood beet greens.**

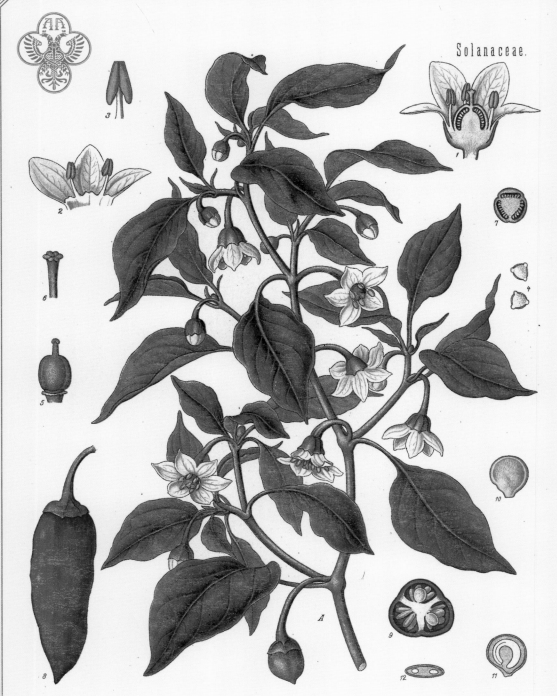

Solanaceae.

Capsicum annuum L.

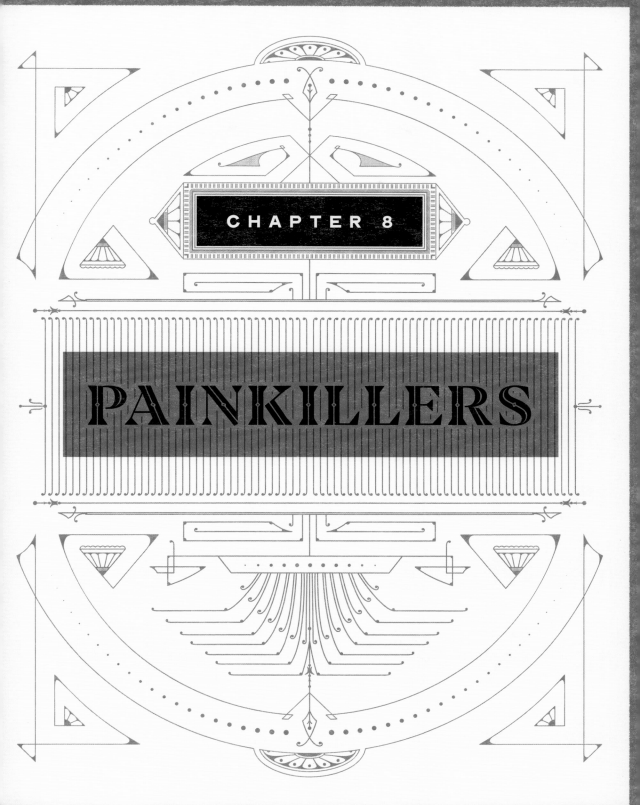

CHAPTER 8

PAINKILLERS

**F**ROM ANCIENT PRACTICES DERIVED FROM PLANTS TO modern synthetic manufacturers, the ability to treat pain is an integral field of medicine. However, it's important to note that alcohol itself is a well-known painkiller. Researchers hypothesize that alcohol blocks the transmission of pain signals in the spinal cord (it is also thought that alcohol's anxiety-relieving properties may play a role). Apotheke uses the benefits of plant science to enhance and expand the inherent pain-inhibiting properties of alcohol.

Pain can be a major quality-of-life killer, and pain relief has become a big business, as well as a controversial one. Apothecaries and physicians used to prescribe several medicines that were later found to be dangerous and addictive. Opium, from the opium poppy plant, was one of the most prescribed drugs in the 1800s. Its products (heroin, laudanum, and morphine) could be purchased over the counter in the United States until 1914, when the Harrison Act was passed, requiring a prescription for narcotics. Laudanum is opium mixed with alcohol, and it is highly addictive. Some of the most notorious laudanum addicts were writers. Paracelsus, the infamous and eccentric Swiss alchemist, first coined the word *laudanum* in the 1500s, and he may have been one of its abusers. Opium and laudanum were even marketed as medicines to quiet and soothe babies. Apothecaries would sell items like elixir of opium.

Other notorious medicines sold in nineteenth-century apothecary shops that have since been proven unsafe include chloroform and strychnine. One must wonder if future societies will similarly identify some of our common medicines as outlandish and dangerous.

Patent medicine makers seized opportunities to market secret mixtures that cured all of your pains. Preparations with a lot of opium and alcohol became popular, and makers didn't have to list their ingredients until the 1906 Pure Food and Drug Act.

## Traits of Ingredients in This Chapter

Habanero peppers belong to the class of peppers that contain capsaicin—a neuropeptide-releasing agent that works by depleting Substance P, a neurotransmitter that transports pain signals to the brain.

Black pepper and ginger also produce a painful irritation. But they relieve pain when painkilling endorphins are released. Black pepper gets its pungency from piperine, which is milder than capsaicin. Ginger has properties that are anti-inflammatory and stomach-soothing. Ancient sage is a powerful healer and anti-inflammatory, as well. Sage boosts cognitive function, and researchers are examining its Alzheimer's disease applications.

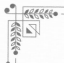

Some early apothecaries treated headaches with vinegar of roses, a remedy made of rose petals steeped in vinegar and applied topically.

## Spirit Notes

Painkillers are all about the whiskey, including bourbon, rye, and Scotch, and occasionally moonshine. Our natural painkillers use the analgesic effects inherent in whiskey, as well as herbs and spices known for their anti-inflammatory and pain-relieving effects.

This section of the menu focuses on formulas that explore the natural pain relief offered by spirts with pain-inhibiting plants.

## FEATURED PAINKILLING BOTANICALS

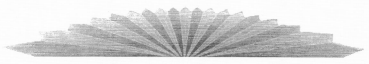

# BLACK PEPPER

# DANDELION ROOT

# EUCALYPTUS

# GINGER

# SAGE

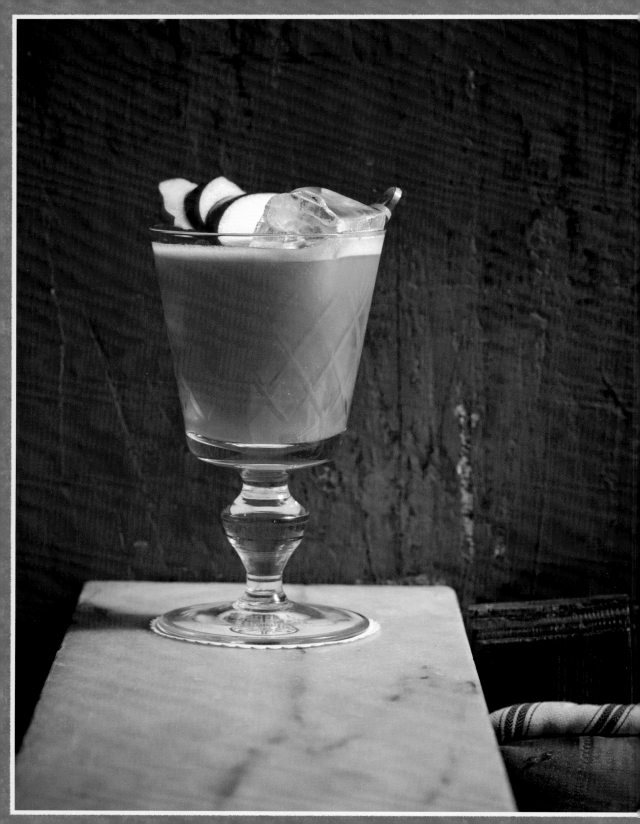

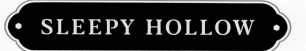

# · SLEEPY HOLLOW ·

*With its apples and butternut squash, Sleepy Hollow is drenched in a New England autumn.*

### FORMULA

3 Granny Smith apple slices,
¼ inch thick

2 ounces bourbon

2 ounces Butternut Squash Purée
*(page 229)*

1 ounce Sour Mix *(page 227)*

Garnish 3 red apple slices

### TOOLS

Muddler

Shaker

Jigger

Hawthorne strainer

Stemmed rocks glass

### EXECUTION

Muddle the Granny Smith apple slices in a shaker. Add the measured
ingredients to the shaker with ice. Shake vigorously. Strain into a stemmed
rocks glass with fresh ice. Garnish with the apple slices.

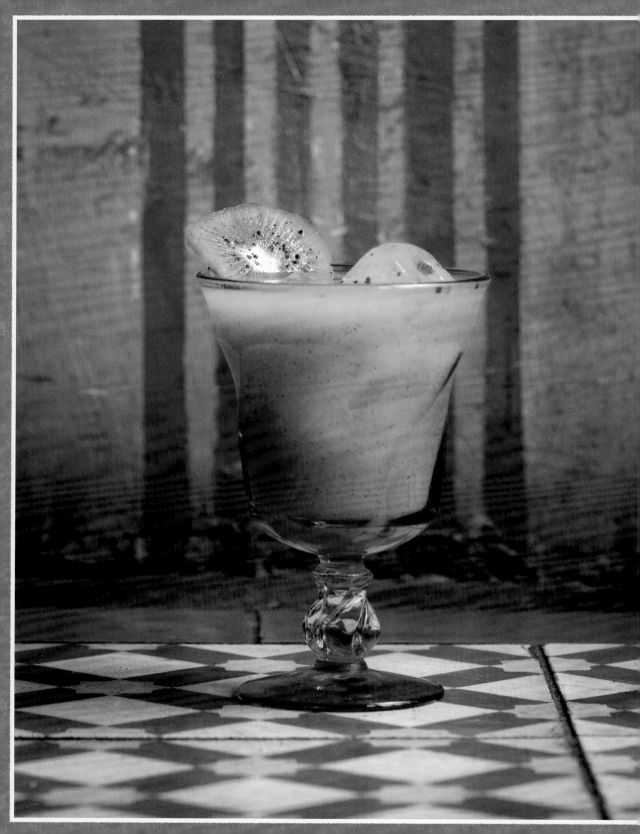

# PYGMY GIMLET

*Eucalyptus-Infused Vodka comes from a land down under, and contrary to its diminutive title, this is a grand gimlet. The initial rush of sweetness from lime and simple syrup is quickly met with the spice of black pepper and then leveled out with the subtle tartness of muddled kiwi. This allows the APO Digestion Bitters to make a triumphant finish.*

## FORMULA

½ kiwi

2 ounces Eucalyptus-Infused Vodka
*(page 233)*

½ ounce lime juice

½ ounce Simple Syrup *(page 226)*

2 cc APO Digestion Bitters
*(recommended)*

2 pinches cracked black pepper

Garnish kiwi slice

## TOOLS

Muddler

Shaker

Jigger

Lemon squeezer

Hawthorne strainer

Stemmed rocks glass

## EXECUTION

**Muddle the kiwi in a shaker. Add the remaining measured ingredients to the shaker with ice and shake vigorously. Strain into a stemmed rocks glass. Crack the pepper over the top of the cocktail. Garnish with a kiwi slice.**

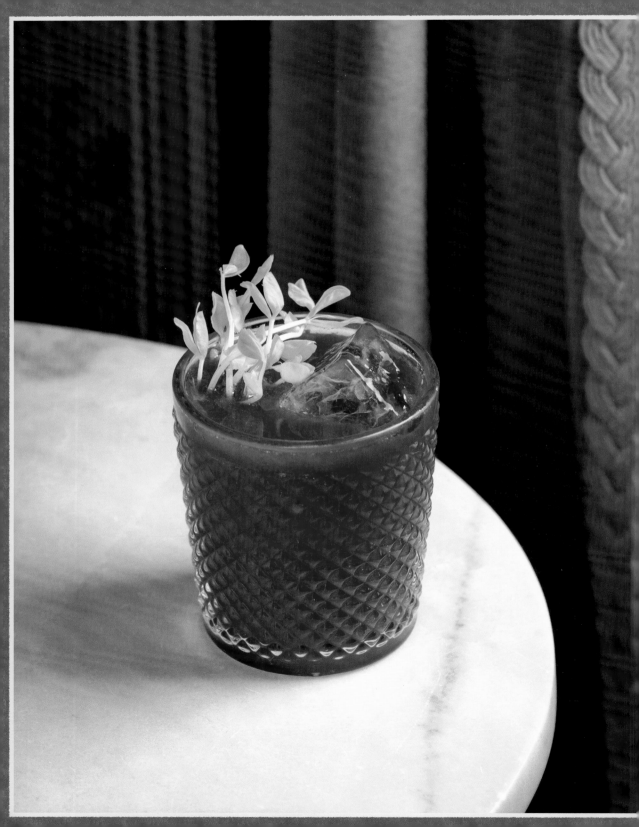

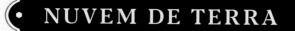

# • NUVEM DE TERRA •

*The storm has begun. Dark, tantalizing flavors spiral in force with rich blackberry açaí and fresh ginger spice, spiked with citrus flavor and then smoothed out with a sweet, seductive rum-and-bourbon blend. All drifted over by a mist of smoky Islay Scotch. Where the earth meets wind.*

## FORMULA

1 ounce bourbon

1 ounce molasses-based rum

1 ounce Blackberry-Açaí Purée
*(page 229)*

¾ ounce Ginger Water *(page 226)*

½ ounce lime juice

½ ounce Simple Syrup *(page 226)*

2 cc APO Immunity Bitters
*(recommended)*

Garnish 3 golden pea shoots

Mist 2 sprays peated Scotch

## TOOLS

Jigger

Lemon squeezer

Shaker

Hawthorne strainer

Rocks glass

Atomizer

## EXECUTION

**Add all of the measured ingredients to a shaker with ice. Shake vigorously. Strain into a rocks glass over fresh ice. Garnish with three golden pea shoots across the top of the rocks glass. Fill the atomizer with peated Scotch and spray twice over the drink.**

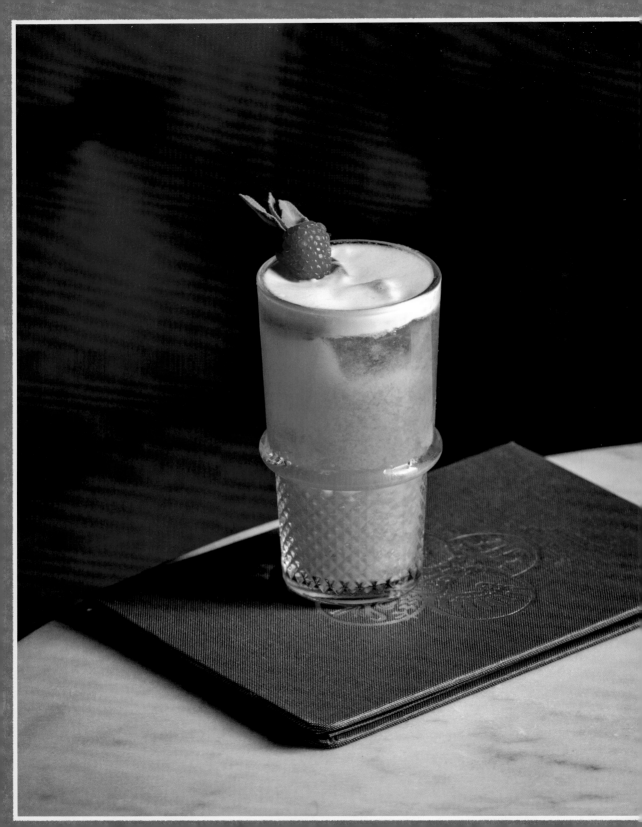

# • WIND BLOSSOM •

*Our attempt to send a classic gin fizz into the sky. Vibrant, tart raspberries and lemon flavor bursts are whipped into balance by the egg white–substitute aquafaba and the botanical prowess of gin. The Wind Blossom is a light, feathery, botanical sour with enough effervescence and froth to float away on.*

## FORMULA

4 raspberries

2 pieces torn sage

2 ounces gin

¼ ounce baijiu

¾ ounce orgeat syrup (*see note*)

¾ ounce lemon juice

½ ounce aquafaba (*see note*)

Top club soda

Garnish raspberry and sage leaf

## TOOLS

Muddler

Shaker

Jigger

Lemon squeezer

Hawthorne strainer

Collins glass

## EXECUTION

**Muddle the raspberries and sage in a shaker. Add the remaining measured ingredients to the shaker with ice. Shake vigorously. Add club soda to the shaker. Strain ingredients into a Collins glass with fresh ice. Garnish with a raspberry and sage leaf.**

NOTE: Orgeat is a sweet syrup made from almonds, sugar, and rose or orange flower water. Aquafaba is readily available for purchase online.

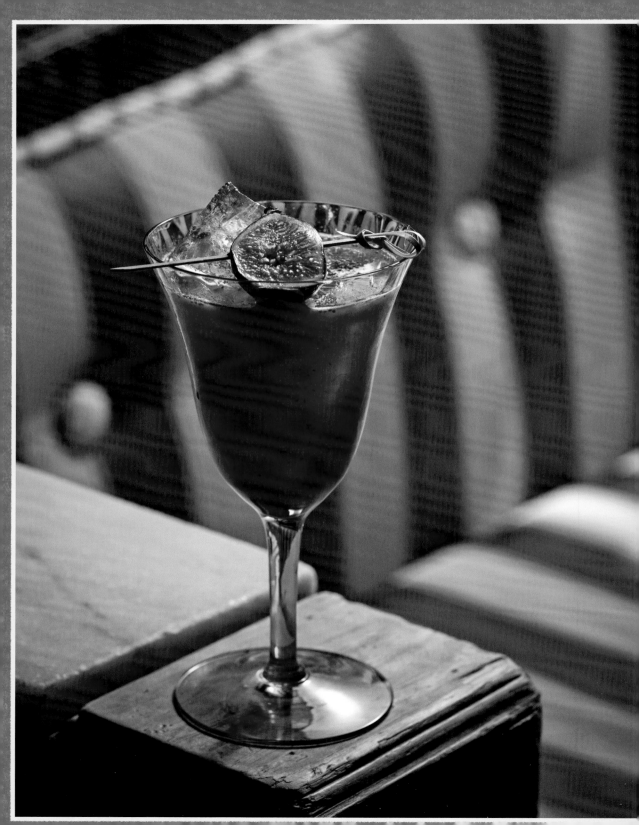

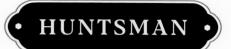

# • HUNTSMAN •

*This is one of our richest drinks. The wintery flavors and the smokiness of the Scotch will transport you to a hunting lodge next to a warm, crackling fire.*

## FORMULA

2 ounces Duck Bacon Fat–Infused Scotch *(page 233)*

1 ounce Fig Purée *(page 229)*

¼ ounce store-bought balsamic glaze

¼ ounce Sour Mix *(page 227)*

Dash Fee Brothers Chocolate Bitters

1 cc APO Immunity Bitters *(recommended)*

Peated Scotch mist

Garnish fig slice

## TOOLS

Jigger

Shaker

Hawthorne strainer

Stemmed glass

Atomizer

## EXECUTION

Add all measured ingredients to a shaker with ice. Shake vigorously. Strain into a stemmed glass over fresh ice. Fill the atomizer with peated Scotch and mist the top of the drink. Garnish with a fig slice.

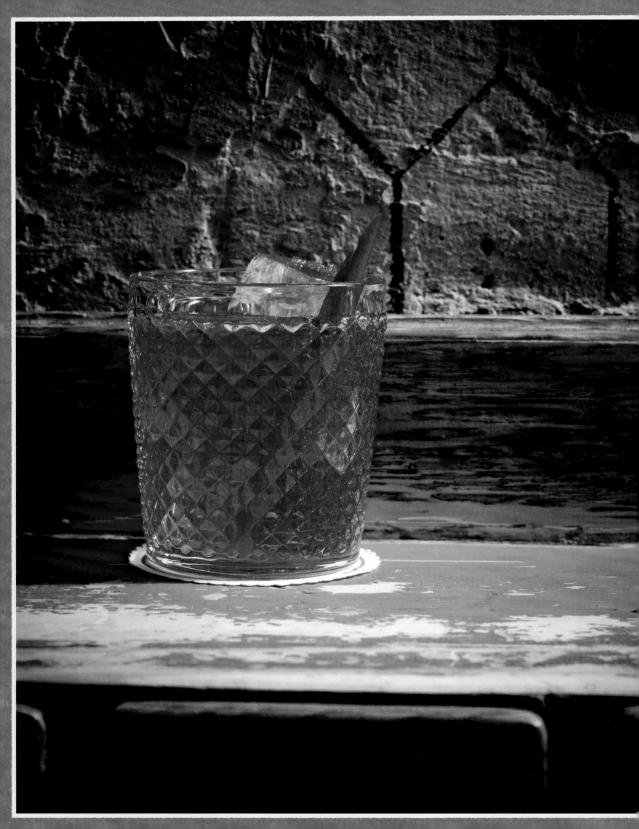

# • PATH OF THE RIGHTEOUS •

*Smoky, oaky, and tart. A herbaceous dive into a deeper, darker take on the boulevardier.
The rhubarb swizzle stick garnish enhances the tartness as you sip and stir.*

## FORMULA

1½ ounces peated Scotch

1 ounce sweet vermouth
(Antica Formula)

¾ ounce Aperol

Bar spoon green chartreuse

Dash Fee Brothers Rhubarb Bitters

Garnish quartered rhubarb
swizzle stick

## TOOLS

Jigger

Mixing glass

Bar spoon

Julep strainer

Rocks glass

## EXECUTION

Add the measured ingredients to a mixing glass with ice. Stir approximately
50 rotations until the liquid is thoroughly chilled. Strain into a rocks glass with
fresh ice. Garnish with rhubarb.

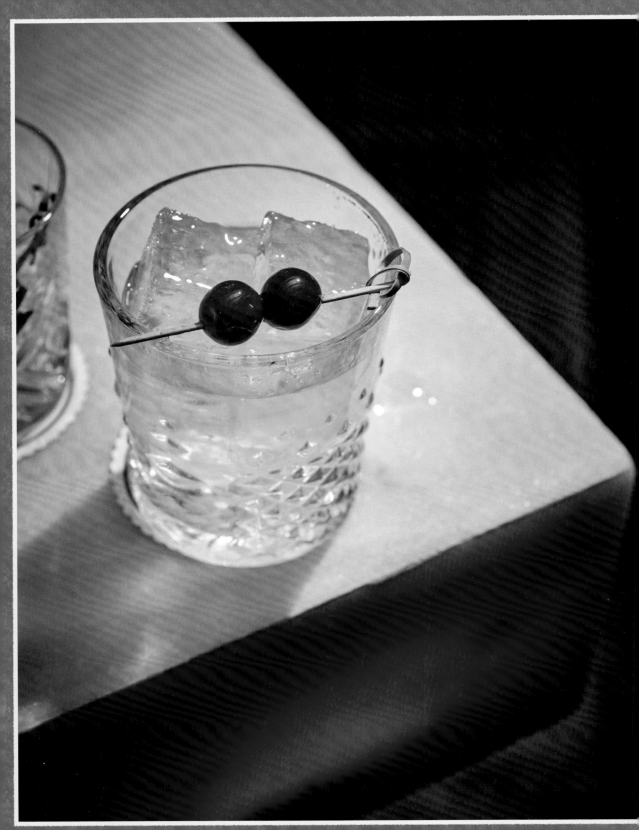

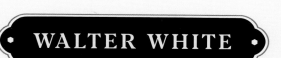

# WALTER WHITE

*Our deceitful take on a classic Manhattan. Corrupted by moonshine and packing serious weight, this stirred poison is sure to start an obsession.*

### FORMULA

2 ounces moonshine

1 ounce *bianco* vermouth

½ ounce Bénédictine

Dash Fee Brothers Grapefruit Bitters

Garnish brandied cherries

### TOOLS

Jigger

Mixing glass

Bar spoon

Julep strainer

Rocks glass

### EXECUTION

Add all measured ingredients to a mixing glass with ice. Stir approximately 50 rotations until the liquid is thoroughly chilled. Strain into a rocks glass with fresh ice. Garnish with 2 brandied cherries.

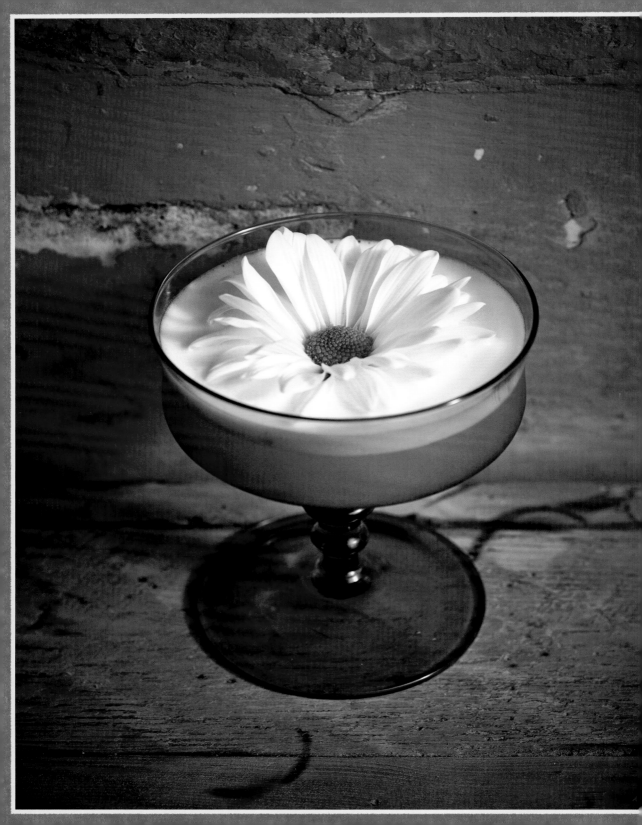

# • A DAISY IF YOU DO •

*This one is earthy but bright with a nod to South America. With its daisy flower garnish, this drink is a visual and olfactory delight.*

## FORMULA

2 ounces Dandelion-Infused Pisco
*(page 232)*

½ ounce Lemon Verbena Simple
Syrup *(page 226)*

½ ounce lemon juice

½ ounce egg white

2 cc APO Digestion Bitters
*(recommended)*

Garnish daisy flower head

## TOOLS

Jigger

Lemon squeezer

Shaker

Hawthorne strainer

Coupe glass

## EXECUTION

**Add all of the measured ingredients to a shaker. Vigorously dry shake
(without ice). Add ice and shake vigorously. Strain into a coupe glass.
Garnish with a daisy.**

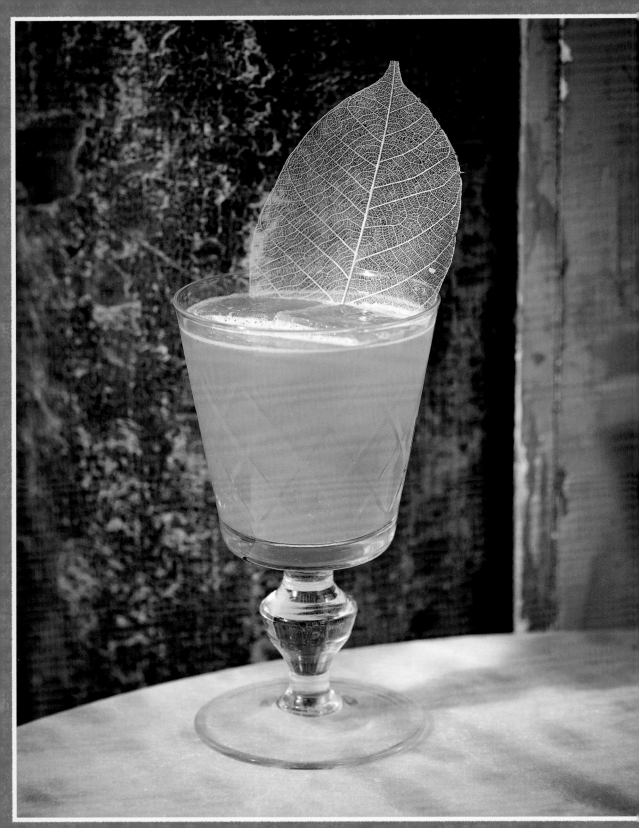

# • DRAGONFLY •

*Spicy, floral, sweet, and complex. The taste of mezcal is nearly nonexistent when infused with sencha tea, which contains dried peach and sunflower blossoms. The epazote leaf adds an exotic touch to a wonderfully eccentric cocktail.*

### FORMULA

Epazote leaf

2 ounces Sencha Tea Mezcal
*(page 234)*

1 ounce Peach Purée *(page 230)*

1 ounce Sour Mix *(page 227)*

¼ ounce Habanero Tincture
*(page 228)*

Garnish skeleton leaf

### TOOLS

Muddler

Shaker

Jigger

Hawthorne strainer

Rocks glass

### EXECUTION

**Muddle the epazote leaf in a shaker. Add all of the measured ingredients to the shaker with ice and shake vigorously. Strain into a rocks glass with fresh ice. Garnish with a skeleton leaf.**

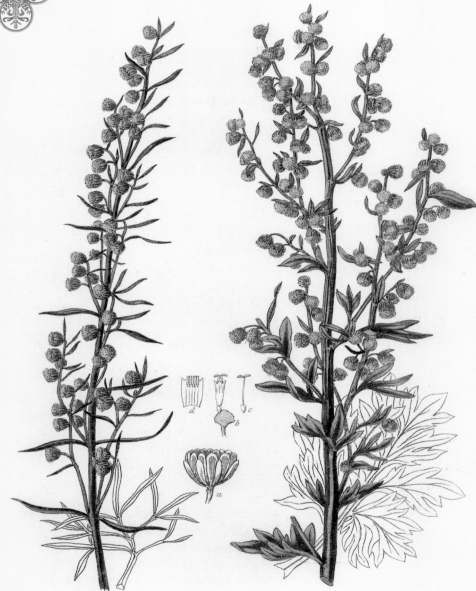

*Artemisia*

*Santonica.*                    *Absinthium.*

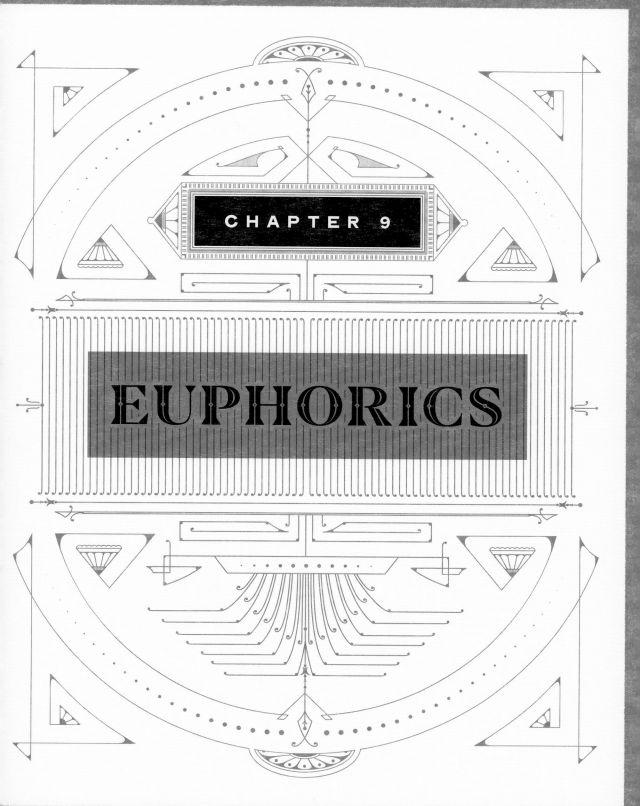

CHAPTER 9

# EUPHORICS

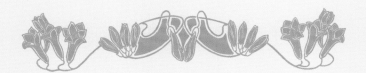

# E
UPHORIA, BEYOND MERE HAPPINESS AND BORDERING
on ecstasy and elation, is a coveted feeling. Alcohol itself gives us a buzz of
euphoria, and we added ingredients to enhance this sense of well-being.

## Traits of Ingredients in This Chapter

Euphoria has an interesting link to pain. The capsaicin in habanero and other peppers is responsible for signaling the brain that something is on fire. The brain responds with pain signals, prompting a fight-or-flight response. But something good also happens: to help the body cope with the burn, the brain produces endorphins. These natural painkillers can lead to a feeling of euphoria.

Matcha is a superfood of the tea world and the go-to tea for Zen Buddhist monks, who use it to stay alert and relaxed during meditation.

Wormwood has been infused in drinks, often wine, for thousands of years for medicinal purposes. Wormwood was listed in the Ebers papyrus—an ancient Egyptian medical scroll from 1500 BCE. (This papyrus is actually believed to encapsulate works from centuries earlier, so the 1500 date is approximate.) The papyrus recommends wormwood for destroying roundworms and soothing digestive issues. Around the same time, the Chinese were making medicinal wines with wormwood. It is the primary ingredient in absinthe.

## Spirit Notes

Some of the drinks in this chapter feature absinthe, which has, for a long time, been associated with a particularly clear-headed, euphoria-inducing feeling. This is one of the absinthe tropes that might actually have some basis in fact: Absinthe's ingredients are a combination of uppers and downers. Alcohol is a central nervous system depressant, but absinthe's herbal constituents have stimulating and serotonin-inducing effects.

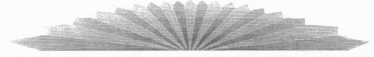

# LAPSANG SOUCHONG

# HABANERO

# MATCHA TEA

# ORANGE BLOSSOM WATER

# WORMWOOD

*Absinthe is the aphrodisiac of the self. The green fairy who lives in the absinthe wants your soul. But you are safe with me.*

—GARY OLDMAN AS DRACULA, *Bram Stoker's Dracula* (1992)

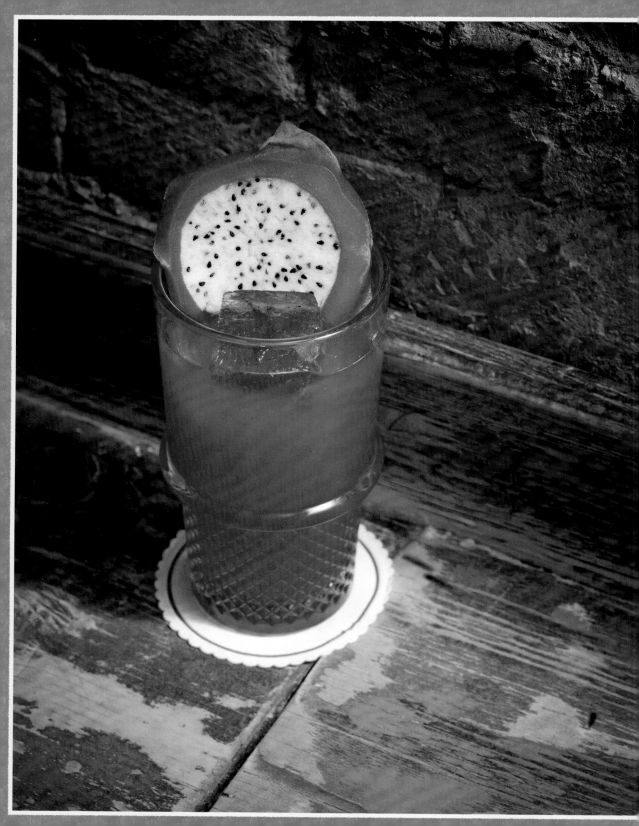

# • DEVIL'S PLAYGROUND •

*Deep, seductive color swirling with earthy botanicals and fruity enticement, all blanketed with the stimulating aroma of anise. The Devil's Playground is a devious concoction that will have the beholder frolicking mischievously through the night.*

## FORMULA

2 ounces gin

1 ounce Prickly Pear–Dragon Fruit Purée *(page 231)*

1 ounce Sour Mix *(page 227)*

2 cc APO Rejuvenation Bitters *(recommended)*

Mist absinthe

Garnish slice of dragon fruit

## TOOLS

Shaker

Jigger

Hawthorne strainer

Collins glass

Atomizer

## EXECUTION

Add all of the measured ingredients to a shaker with ice. Shake vigorously. Strain into a Collins glass with fresh ice. Fill the atomizer with absinthe and mist over the glass. Garnish with dragon fruit.

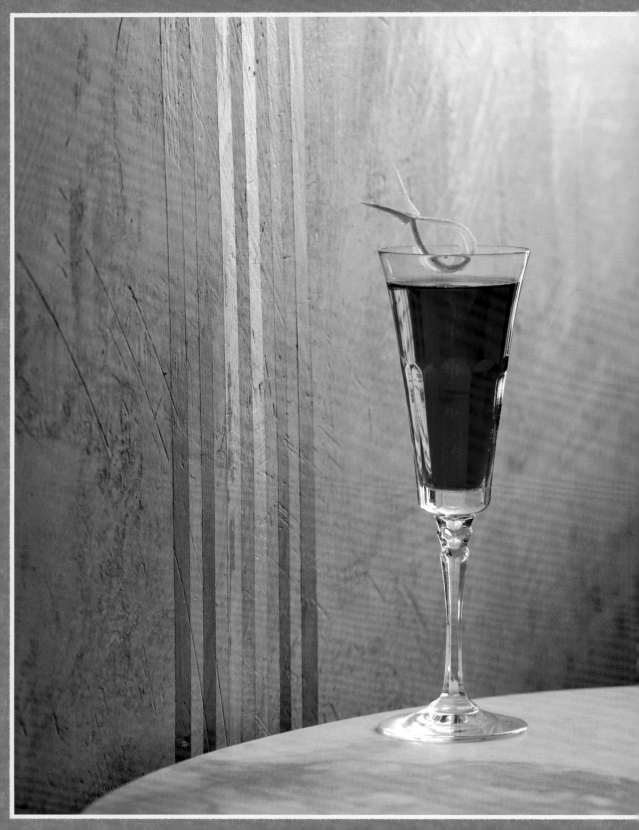

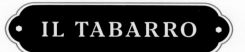

# • IL TABARRO •

*The Italian* il tabarro *translates to "the cloak." This cocktail is a smoky take on the classic Negroni that wraps you up in all its dark botanical glory and then sends you off into the night.*

## FORMULA

2 ounces Lapsang Souchong
Tea-Infused Gin *(page 233)*

1 ounce Aperol

1 ounce Carpano Antica Formula
*(sweet vermouth)*

Garnish blood orange peel

## TOOLS

Jigger

Mixing glass

Bar spoon

Julep strainer

Stemmed glass

Citrus peeler

## EXECUTION

**Add all the measured ingredients to a mixing glass. Add ice and stir approximately 50 rotations until the liquid is thoroughly chilled. Strain into a stemmed glass. Garnish with blood orange peel.**

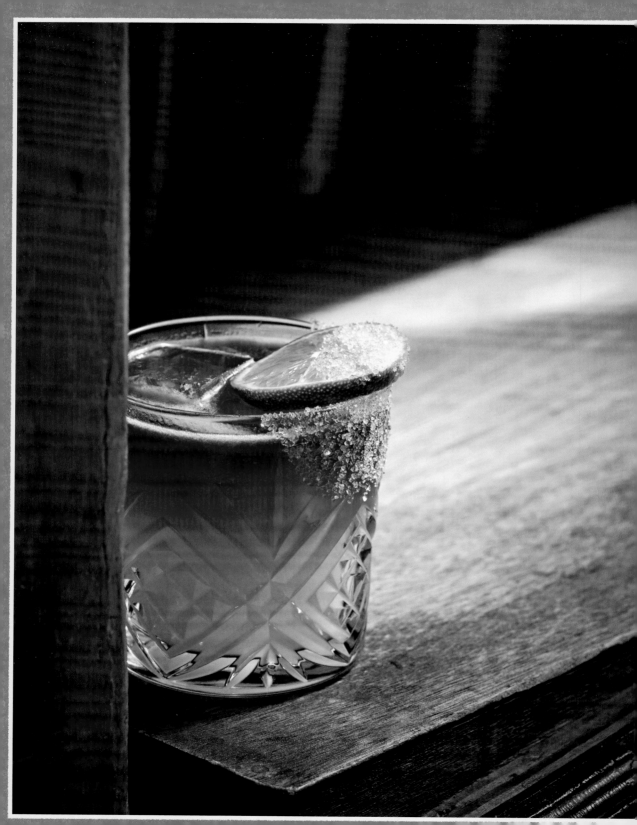

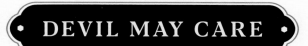

# · DEVIL MAY CARE ·

*Take the classic margarita and give it a sophisticated, beautiful twist with pink Himalayan salt and a cabernet floater.*

## FORMULA

2 ounces tequila

½ ounce Cointreau

¾ ounce Ginger Mix *(page 226)*

1 ounce Sour Mix *(page 227)*

2 shakes orange blossom water

Orange wedge

Rim pink Himalayan sea salt

Cabernet

Garnish pink Himalayan–salted
lime wheel

## TOOLS

Jigger

Shaker

Hawthorne strainer

Rocks glass

Bar spoon

## EXECUTION

Add all measured ingredients to a shaker with ice. Shake vigorously.
Rub the rim of a rocks glass with an orange wedge, rim the glass with Himalayan
sea salt, and fill it with fresh ice. Strain the cocktail into the rocks glass and float
the wine (see page 161) using a bar spoon. Garnish with the salted lime wheel.

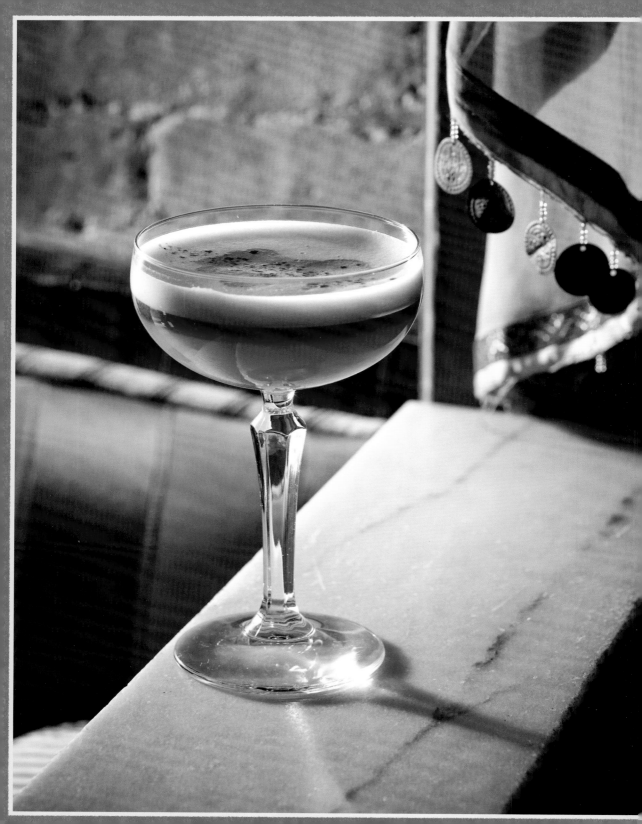

# • TOKYO DRIFT •

*Where Asia meets Kentucky. This is our take on a bourbon sour, but soaked with matcha tea and cabernet. The diverse ingredients create an impressive visual layering.*

### FORMULA

1½ ounces bourbon
½ ounce sake
1 ounce matcha tea
1 ounce Sour Mix *(page 227)*
½ ounce egg white
Cabernet
Garnish matcha powder

### TOOLS

Jigger
Shaker
Hawthorne strainer
Coupe glass
Bar spoon

### EXECUTION

Add all of the measured ingredients to a shaker. Dry shake (without ice).
Add ice and shake vigorously. Strain into a coupe glass. Using the bar spoon,
float a small layer of cabernet (see page 161) on the top. It should settle beneath
the egg white foam and above the other liquid. Garnish with matcha powder.

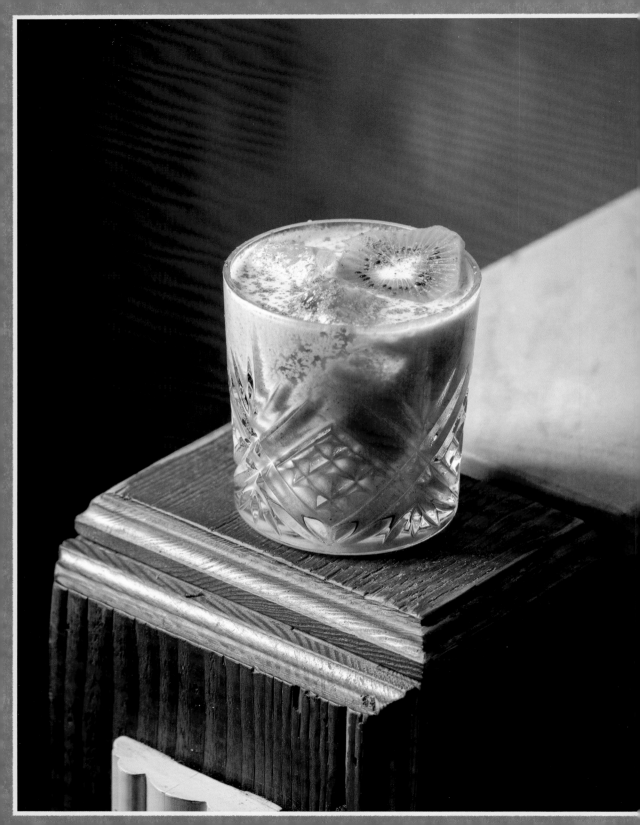

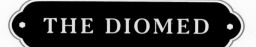

# · THE DIOMED ·

*Taking far-flung ingredients from around the world and drawing influences from classic*
*tiki recipes, this is an amazingly vibrant cocktail. Generally, this many bold flavors would*
*stomp all over one another and create unbalanced chaos. But the Diomed's precise layers*
*present its special ingredients in a sophisticated light. All the flavors work in unison*
*to create a balanced and bright cocktail experience. Tart, sweet, and creamy, there's a*
*different flavor to grab hold of in every sip.*

### FORMULA

2 pieces blood orange

2 ounces bourbon

¾ ounce Kiwi-Pandan Purée *(page 230)*

½ ounce heavy cream

½ ounce Simple Syrup *(page 226)*

¼ ounce lime juice

Garnish kiwi slice

Garnish ground allspice

### TOOLS

Muddler

Shaker

Jigger

Lemon squeezer

Hawthorne strainer

Rocks glass

### EXECUTION

**Muddle the blood orange in a shaker. Add all of the measured ingredients to the**
**shaker with ice. Shake vigorously. Strain the ingredients into a rocks glass over**
**fresh ice. Garnish with a kiwi slice and sprinkle ground allspice over the top.**

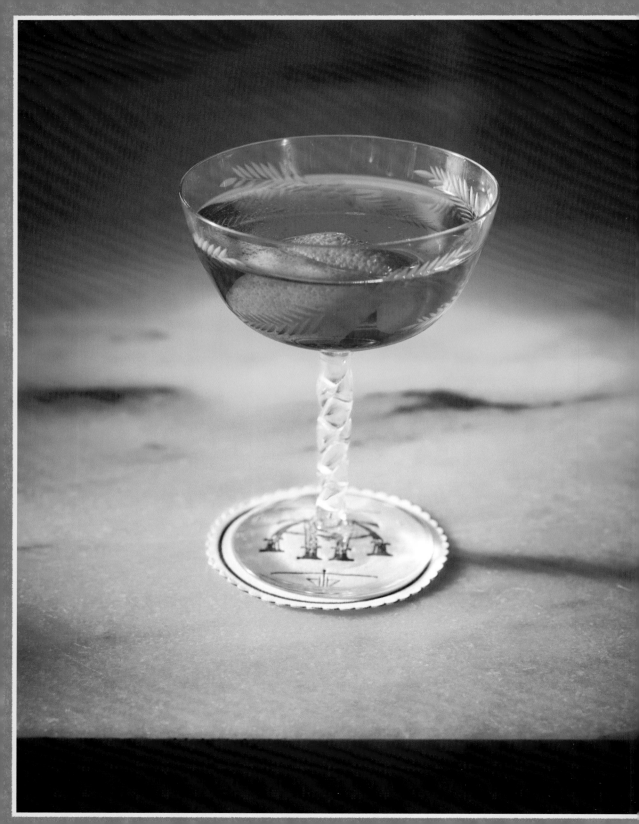

# • HIGH PLAINS DRIFTER •

*The High Plains Drifter is a take on a classic—the Sazerac—with a key difference:*
*Barley-Infused Rye. An infusion being almost like a reverse marinade, we let the liquid*
*take on the character of the solid. The toasted barley amplifies and complements the*
*bite and earthiness of the rye, which gives this cocktail a memorable finish. A light citrus*
*zest and an absinthe rinse are finished with a sparkle of sarsaparilla powder, giving the*
*cocktail a versatile nose.*

### FORMULA

3 ounces Barley-Infused Rye
*(page 232)*
Dash Peychaud's Bitters
Dollop agave nectar
¼ ounce absinthe
3 pinches sarsaparilla powder
Garnish orange peel

### TOOLS

Jigger
Mixing glass
Bar spoon
Coupe glass
Lighter
Julep strainer
Citrus peeler

### EXECUTION

Add the rye, bitters, and nectar to a mixing glass with ice and stir approximately
50 rotations, until the liquid is thoroughly chilled. Roll the absinthe around the
inside of a coupe glass, light it, and sprinkle sarsaparilla powder into the flame,
to create sparkles. Discard any remaining absinthe. Strain the mixing glass into
the coupe glass. Garnish with an orange peel.

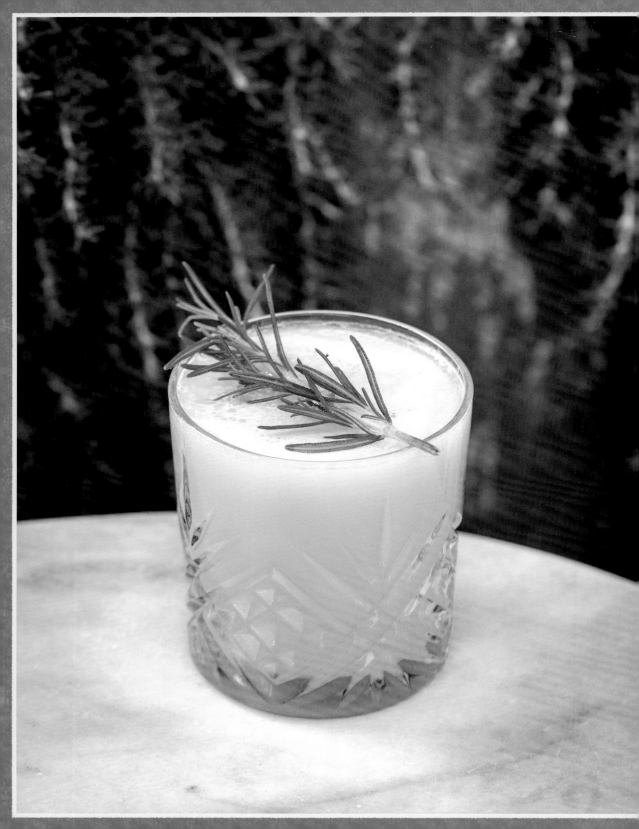

# LAND WAR IN ASIA

*Despite how explosive this Far East–inspired cocktail's ingredients may sound, the delicately balanced blend of teas and citrus flow seamlessly together, with a soft texture created by the addition of aquafaba and a botanical spirit base. Having the flavor and nutritional driving force from fresh tea is an amazing way to subtly invigorate your drink. Top that off with a burst of flaming rosemary to bring back a stark, pungent, chaotic element. This cocktail truly tells a story through liquid.*

### FORMULA

2 ounces gin

½ ounce matcha tea

¾ ounce royal milk tea *(see note)*

½ ounce aquafaba *(see note)*

½ ounce lime juice

½ ounce Simple Syrup *(page 226)*

Garnish absinthe-soaked
rosemary sprig

### TOOLS

Jigger

Lemon squeezer

Shaker

Hawthorne strainer

Rocks glass

Lighter

### EXECUTION

**Place all of the measured ingredients into a shaker with ice. Shake vigorously (the aquafaba needs to froth). Strain into a rocks glass over fresh ice. Dip the rosemary sprig into absinthe, light the rosemary, and place it on top of the rocks glass. Extinguish rosemary sprig before consuming the cocktail.**

NOTE: Royal milk tea and aquafaba are readily available for purchase online.

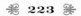

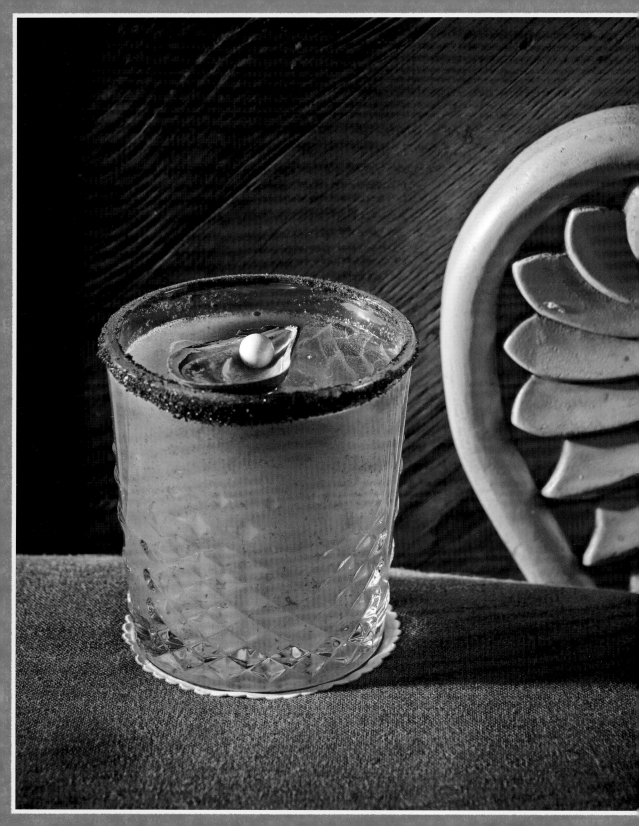

# • SIREN'S CALL •

*One of the most ambitious and unusual cocktails on the menu, the Siren's Call began with the idea to do a nautical-themed drink. The proper technique for drinking this cocktail is to roll the pearl into your mouth, then take the shell and drop it into your drink. The shell adds just a bit more of that salty, ocean-y flavor and texture to the drink.*

### FORMULA

2 ounces gin

1 ounce Cucumber–Seaweed Purée
*(page 229)*

¾ ounce Ginger Mix *(page 226)*

¾ ounce Sour Mix *(page 227)*

2 drops squid ink

2 cc APO Illuminate Bitters
*(recommended)*

Orange slice

Rim black lava salt

Garnish mussel shell and
candy pearl

### TOOLS

Jigger

Shaker

Rocks glass

Hawthorne strainer

### EXECUTION

**Place all of the measured ingredients into a shaker with ice. Shake vigorously. Rub the rim of the rocks glass with an orange slice and rim the glass with black lava salt. Strain the cocktail into the glass with fresh ice. Garnish with a mussel shell and candy pearl.**

# COMPENDIUM

*Recipes with specified quantities make enough for at least 4 cocktails.*
*We recommend using a digital food scale for weighing.*

## BASICS

### GINGER MIX

200 GRAMS GINGER ROOT
1 OUNCE LIME JUICE
1 OUNCE SIMPLE SYRUP *(below)*

Peel, then cut the ginger root into ½-inch chunks. Place the ginger root, lime juice, and simple syrup into a blender and blend until liquified. Pour the mixture through a chinois strainer into a clean, airtight glass container. Discard the fibrous material. Store in the refrigerator.

### GINGER WATER

150 GRAMS GINGER ROOT

Cover the ginger root in water and let it soak overnight at room temperature; discard the water. Peel the ginger and run it through a juicer. Add equal parts water to the ginger juice. Strain the mixture through a chinois strainer into a clean, airtight glass container. Discard the fibrous material.

### LEMON VERBENA SIMPLE SYRUP

4 OUNCES WATER
1 GRAM LEMON VERBENA LEAVES
100 GRAMS GRANULATED SUGAR

Place the water in a small saucepan set over low heat. Allow the water to heat until it's just under boiling point and then remove from the heat. Add the lemon verbena leaves and steep for 5 minutes. Strain out the lemon verbena leaves; discard the leaves. Add the sugar and steeped tea to a sealable container and agitate until the sugar dissolves. Transfer to a clean, airtight glass container and refrigerate.

### SIMPLE SYRUP

1 PART GRANULATED SUGAR
1 PART WATER

Place the sugar and water in a small saucepan set over medium heat. Stir until the sugar dissolves. Let cool, then store in a clean, airtight glass container.

## HEAVY SIMPLE SYRUP

2 PARTS GRANULATED SUGAR
1 PART WATER

Place the sugar and water in a small saucepan set over medium heat. Stir until the sugar dissolves. Let cool, then store in a clean, airtight glass container.

## SOUR MIX

1 PART LIME JUICE
1 PART HEAVY SIMPLE syrup
*(previous recipe)*

Combine the lime juice and heavy simple syrup in a clean, airtight glass container. Stir and store in refrigerator.

## CORDIALS

### ANCHO CHILI CORDIAL

8 OUNCES (1 CUP) VODKA
1½ OUNCES PEATED SCOTCH
20 GRAMS ANCHO CHILIES
¾ GRAM CINNAMON STICK
50 GRAMS GRANULATED SUGAR

In a small bowl, combine the vodka, Scotch, and ancho chilies and let sit at room temperature for 90 minutes. Add the cinnamon stick and let the mixture sit for an additional 90 minutes. Strain into a small saucepan and discard the chilies and cinnamon stick. Add the sugar to the saucepan and stir over low heat until the sugar is completely dissolved. Do not allow it to boil. Let cool, then store in a clean, airtight glass container.

### HONEY-CHAMOMILE CORDIAL

8 OUNCES (1 CUP) RYE WHISKEY
6 GRAMS BLACK PEPPERCORNS
5 GRAMS CHAMOMILE FLOWERS
2 OUNCES HONEY

In a small bowl, combine the rye whiskey with the black peppercorns and chamomile flowers. Let sit for 3½ hours at room temperature. Strain with

a chinois strainer into a medium bowl; discard the solids. Add the honey and mix thoroughly. Store in a clean, airtight glass container.

### ORANGE CORDIAL

8 OUNCES (1 CUP) VODKA
10 GRAMS ORANGE RIND
40 GRAMS RAW CANE SUGAR
¼ OUNCE ORANGE BLOSSOM WATER

In a measuring cup, steep the vodka with the orange rind until a strong orange flavor develops, about 6 hours. Remove the orange rind and discard. Place the orange-infused vodka into a small saucepan set over low heat and add the cane sugar, stirring to dissolve. Do not allow it to boil. Let cool, add the orange blossom water, and transfer to a clean, airtight glass container.

### LAVENDER CORDIAL

8 OUNCES (1 CUP) VODKA
10 GRAMS ORANGE RIND
3 GRAMS LAVENDER BUDS
40 GRAMS RAW CANE SUGAR
¼ OUNCE ORANGE BLOSSOM WATER

In a measuring cup, steep the vodka with the orange rind for 3 hours. Add the lavender buds. Let sit for an additional 3 hours. Strain the vodka into a small saucepan; discard the orange rind and

lavender. Warm the vodka over low heat, then add the cane sugar, stirring to dissolve. Do not allow it to boil. Let cool, add the orange blossom water, and transfer to a clean, airtight glass container.

## SHRUB

### POMEGRANATE SHRUB

8 CUPS POMEGRANATE CONCENTRATE
2 CUPS SIMPLE SYRUP (page 226)
3 OUNCES BALSAMIC VINEGAR

Mix all ingredients together. Store in a clean, airtight glass container and keep refrigerated.

## TINCTURES

### BILBERRY TINCTURE

4 OUNCES (½ CUP) VODKA
3 GRAMS DRIED BILBERRY LEAF

In a measuring cup, steep the vodka with the bilberry leaf for 6 hours. Pour through a chinois strainer into a clean, airtight glass container.

### HABANERO TINCTURE

4 OUNCES (½ CUP) VODKA
8 GRAMS HABANERO PEPPERS

Pour the vodka into a measuring cup. Cut habanero peppers into small pieces and remove all seeds. Place the peppers into the vodka and let sit for 6 hours. Pour through a chinois strainer into a clean, airtight glass container.

### HIBISCUS TINCTURE

4 OUNCES (½ CUP) VODKA
3½ GRAMS DRIED HIBISCUS FLOWER

Pour the vodka into a measuring cup. Place the dried hibiscus flower in the vodka and let sit for 1 hour. Pour through a chinois strainer into a clean, airtight glass container.

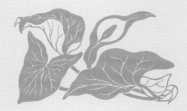

## PURÉES

### BLACKBERRY-AÇAÍ PURÉE

120 GRAMS BLACKBERRIES
33 GRAMS FROZEN AÇAÍ
¼ OUNCE LIME JUICE
¼ OUNCE SIMPLE SYRUP *(page 226)*

Add all the ingredients to a blender and blend until smooth. Store in a clean, airtight glass container and keep refrigerated.

### BLUEBERRY–DRAGON FRUIT PURÉE

100 GRAMS DRAGON FRUIT
2 OUNCES BLUEBERRY JUICE
¼ OUNCE LIME JUICE
¼ OUNCE SIMPLE SYRUP *(page 226)*

Cut the dragon fruit lengthwise, scoop out the fruit, and add to a blender with the other ingredients. Blend until smooth. Store in a clean, airtight glass container and keep refrigerated.

### BUTTERNUT SQUASH PURÉE

175 GRAMS BUTTERNUT SQUASH
0.8 GRAM GROUND ALLSPICE
0.4 GRAM GROUND CLOVE

Preheat the oven to 400°F. Cut the squash in half and remove the seeds, then cut into cubes. Roast the cubes for 20 minutes. Once cool, place the cubes in a blender. Blend all ingredients until smooth. Store in a clean, airtight glass container and keep refrigerated.

### CANTALOUPE PURÉE

200 GRAMS CANTALOUPE, CUBED
¼ OUNCE LIME JUICE
¼ OUNCE SIMPLE SYRUP *(page 226)*

Add all ingredients to a blender and blend until smooth. Strain into a clean, airtight glass container; discard seeds. Keep refrigerated.

### CANTALOUPE-BANANA PURÉE

100 GRAMS CANTALOUPE, SEEDED AND CUBED
21 GRAMS BANANA
¼ OUNCE LIME JUICE
¼ OUNCE SIMPLE SYRUP *(page 226)*

Add all ingredients to a blender and blend until smooth. Strain into a clean, airtight glass container; discard seeds. Keep refrigerated.

### CUCUMBER-SEAWEED PURÉE

150 GRAMS ENGLISH (SEEDLESS) CUCUMBER
½ GRAM ROASTED SEAWEED

Add ingredients to a blender and blend until smooth. Store in a clean, airtight glass container and keep refrigerated.

### FIG PURÉE

225 GRAMS TURKISH FIGS
¼ OUNCE LIME JUICE
¼ OUNCE SIMPLE SYRUP *(page 226)*

Add all ingredients to a blender and blend until smooth. Store in a clean, airtight glass container and keep refrigerated.

### GUAVA–BLOOD ORANGE PURÉE

225 GRAMS PEELED GUAVA
1½ OUNCES BLOOD ORANGE JUICE

Add ingredients to a blender and blend until smooth. Store in a clean, airtight glass container and keep refrigerated.

### HONEYDEW PURÉE

300 GRAMS HONEYDEW MELON, CUBED

Add melon to a blender and blend until smooth. Strain into a clean, airtight glass container; discard seeds. Keep refrigerated.

### HONEYDEW-SPIRULINA PURÉE

300 GRAMS HONEYDEW MELON, CUBED
2 GRAMS SPIRULINA POWDER

Add ingredients to a blender and blend until smooth. Strain into a clean, airtight glass container; discard seeds. Keep refrigerated.

### KALE-PINEAPPLE PURÉE

100 GRAMS PINEAPPLE, CUBED
¾ OUNCE KALE JUICE
¼ OUNCE LIME JUICE
¼ OUNCE SIMPLE SYRUP *(page 226)*

Add all ingredients to a blender and blend until smooth. Store in a clean, airtight glass container and keep refrigerated.

### KIWI-PANDAN PURÉE

8 KIWIS, PEELED AND CUBED
8 OUNCES PANDAN JELLY

Blend the ingredients until smooth. Store in a clean, airtight glass container and refrigerate.

### MANGO LASSI PURÉE

150 GRAMS MANGO, CUBED
1½ OUNCES GOAT'S MILK YOGURT

Add ingredients to a blender and blend until smooth. Store in a clean, airtight glass container and keep refrigerated.

### NECTARINE-GOLDEN BEET PURÉE

150 GRAMS NECTARINE
2 OUNCES GOLDEN BEET JUICE
½ OUNCE SIMPLE SYRUP *(page 226)*

Add all ingredients to a blender and blend until smooth. Store in a clean, airtight glass container and keep refrigerated.

### PASSION FRUIT PURÉE

200 GRAMS PASSION FRUIT

Cut passion fruit lengthwise and scoop out pulp and seeds in a blender with 1 tablespoon water. Blend until smooth. Strain into a clean, airtight glass container; discard seeds. Keep refrigerated.

### PEACH PURÉE

225 GRAMS PEACHES
½ OUNCE WHEATGRASS JUICE
½ OUNCE LIME JUICE
¼ OUNCE SIMPLE SYRUP *(page 226)*

Add all ingredients to a blender and blend until smooth. Store in a clean, airtight glass container and keep refrigerated.

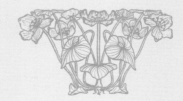

## PINEAPPLE PURÉE

200 GRAMS PINEAPPLE, CUBED
¼ OUNCE LIME
¼ OUNCE SIMPLE SYRUP *(page 226)*

Add all ingredients to a blender and blend until smooth. Store in a clean, airtight glass container and keep refrigerated.

## PLUM-CARDAMOM PURÉE

200 GRAMS RED PLUMS
1 GRAM GROUND CARDAMOM
¼ OUNCE LIME JUICE
¼ OUNCE SIMPLE SYRUP *(page 226)*

Add all ingredients to a blender and blend until smooth. Store in a clean, airtight glass container and keep refrigerated.

## PRICKLY PEAR PURÉE

200 GRAMS PRICKLY PEAR, PEELED
¼ OUNCE LIME JUICE
½ OUNCE SIMPLE SYRUP *(page 226)*

Add all ingredients to a blender and blend until smooth. Strain into a clean, airtight glass container; discard seeds. Keep refrigerated.

## PRICKLY PEAR-DRAGON FRUIT PURÉE

175 GRAMS PRICKLY PEAR, PEELED
75 GRAMS DRAGON FRUIT

Add prickly pear to a blender and blend until smooth. Strain into a bowl; discard seeds. Return the prickly pear to the blender. Cut the dragon fruit lengthwise and scoop out the fruit. Add it to the blender. Blend until smooth. Store in a clean, airtight glass container and keep refrigerated.

## SHISO-TARO ROOT PURÉE

4 CUPS WHOLE TARO ROOT
15 SHISO LEAVES

In a blender, process the taro root and shiso leaves together until smooth. Store in a clean, airtight glass container and refrigerate.

## STRAWBERRY PURÉE

130 GRAMS STRAWBERRIES
1 GRAM ROSEMARY LEAVES
¼ OUNCE ALOE VERA JUICE

Add all ingredients to a blender and blend until smooth. Store in a clean, airtight glass container and keep refrigerated.

## STRAWBERRY, WATERMELON, *and* ARUGULA PURÉE

60 GRAMS WATERMELON, CUBED
60 GRAMS STRAWBERRIES
2 GRAMS ARUGULA
¼ OUNCE LIME JUICE
¼ OUNCE SIMPLE SYRUP *(page 226)*

Add all ingredients to a blender and blend until smooth. Store in a clean, airtight glass container and keep refrigerated.

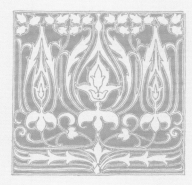

## INFUSIONS

### ACTIVATED CHARCOAL–INFUSED VODKA

8 OUNCES (1 CUP) VODKA
2 GRAMS ACTIVATED CHARCOAL POWDER

Pour the vodka into a measuring cup. Add the activated charcoal and stir until the color of the mixture is black. Store in a clean, airtight glass container. Agitate before each use.

### BARLEY-INFUSED RYE

8 OUNCES (1 CUP) RYE WHISKEY
4 GRAMS TOASTED BARLEY

Pour the rye into a measuring cup. Add the barley to the rye and let sit for 3 hours. Pour through a strainer into a clean, airtight glass container.

### BASIL-INFUSED MEZCAL

8 OUNCES (1 CUP) MEZCAL
7 GRAMS BASIL

Pour the mezcal into a measuring cup. Add the basil leaves to the mezcal and let sit for 12 hours. Strain into a clean, airtight glass container.

### BEET-INFUSED GIN

8 OUNCES (1 CUP) GIN
20 GRAMS BEETS, FINELY CUBED

Pour the gin into a measuring cup. Add the beet cubes to the gin. Let sit for 3 hours. Strain into a clean, airtight glass container.

### BUDDHA'S HAND–INFUSED GIN

8 OUNCES (1 CUP) GIN
20 GRAMS BUDDHA'S HAND, THINLY SLICED

Pour the gin into a measuring cup. Place the Buddha's Hand slices into the gin. Let sit for 8 hours. Strain into a clean, airtight glass container.

### CILANTRO-INFUSED TEQUILA

8 OUNCES (1 CUP) TEQUILA BLANCO
8 GRAMS CILANTRO SPRIGS

Pour the tequila into a measuring cup. Place the cilantro into the tequila. Let sit for 14 hours. Strain into a clean, airtight glass container.

### COFFEE-INFUSED SCOTCH

8 OUNCES (1 CUP) SCOTCH
4 GRAMS GROUND DARK ROAST COFFEE BEANS

Pour the Scotch into a measuring cup. Add the ground coffee to the Scotch. Let sit for 2 hours. Strain into a clean, airtight glass container.

### DANDELION-INFUSED PISCO

8 OUNCES (1 CUP) PISCO
1¾ GRAMS DRIED DANDELION ROOT LOOSE TEA

Pour the pisco into a measuring cup. Add the dandelion root to the pisco. Let infuse for 3 hours. Strain into a clean, airtight glass container.

### DUCK BACON FAT-INFUSED SCOTCH

8 OUNCES (1 CUP) SCOTCH
4 SLICES STORE-BOUGHT DUCK BACON

Cook the duck bacon and render the fat. Pour the Scotch into a measuring cup and add ¾ ounces of the liquid fat into the Scotch. Mix the fat into the scotch, pour the mixture into a freezer-safe container, then freeze overnight. The fat will solidify and form a layer at the top; remove and discard the fat. Store the Scotch in a clean, airtight glass container and keep refrigerated.

### ESPRESSO, BLACK WALNUT HUSK, *and* ALLSPICE-INFUSED BOURBON

8 OUNCES (1 CUP) BOURBON
2½ GRAMS BLACK WALNUT HUSKS
7 GRAMS GROUND COFFEE BEANS
6 GRAMS GROUND ALLSPICE

Pour the bourbon into a measuring cup. Place the black walnut husks into the bourbon. Let sit for 2 hours. Add the coffee and allspice. Let sit for an additional 2 hours. Strain into a clean, airtight glass container.

### EUCALYPTUS-INFUSED VODKA

8 OUNCES (1 CUP) VODKA
1 GRAM DRIED EUCALYPTUS LEAF

Pour the vodka into a measuring cup. Add the eucalyptus to the vodka. Let sit for 3 hours. Strain into a clean, airtight glass container.

### JASMINE TEA *and* SAKE-INFUSED VODKA

5 OUNCES VODKA
3¾ OUNCES SAKE
2 GRAMS JASMINE TEA LEAVES

Mix all the ingredients together in a measuring cup. Let sit for 2 hours. Strain into a clean, airtight glass container.

### LAPSANG SOUCHONG TEA-INFUSED GIN

8 OUNCES (1 CUP) GIN
5 GRAMS LAPSANG SOUCHONG TEA LEAVES

Pour the gin into a measuring cup. Add the tea to the gin. Let sit for 2 hours. Strain into a clean, airtight glass container.

### LAVENDER-INFUSED VODKA

8 OUNCES (1 CUP) VODKA
2 GRAMS LAVENDER BUDS

Pour the vodka into a measuring cup. Add the lavender to the vodka. Let sit for 12 hours. Strain into a clean, airtight glass container.

### LEMONGRASS-INFUSED VODKA

8 OUNCES (1 CUP) VODKA
16 GRAMS LEMONGRASS SHOOTS

Pour the vodka into a measuring cup. Halve the lemongrass lengthwise and add to the vodka. Let sit for 6 hours. Strain into a clean, airtight glass container.

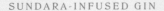

## MACA-INFUSED RUM

8 OUNCES (1 CUP) RUM
2 GRAMS MACA POWDER

Pour the rum into a measuring cup. Add the maca powder to the rum and lightly agitate. Store in a clean, airtight glass container.

## MILK THISTLE–INFUSED VODKA

8 OUNCES (1 CUP) VODKA
2 GRAMS MILK THISTLE TEA

Pour the vodka into a measuring cup. Add the milk thistle tea to the vodka. Let sit for 3 hours. Strain into a clean, airtight glass container.

## ROSEMARY-INFUSED VODKA

8 OUNCES (1 CUP) VODKA
2 GRAMS CUT ROSEMARY SPRIGS

Pour the vodka into a measuring cup. Add the rosemary sprigs to the vodka. Let sit for 4 hours. Strain into a clean, airtight glass container.

## SENCHA TEA MEZCAL

8 OUNCES (1 CUP) MEZCAL
3 GRAMS SENCHA GREEN TEA LEAVES
3 GRAMS SUNFLOWER BLOSSOMS
7½ GRAMS ORGANIC DRIED PEACHES

Combine all ingredients in a measuring cup. Let sit for 4 hours. Strain into a clean, airtight glass container.

## SUNDARA-INFUSED GIN

8 OUNCES (1 CUP) GIN
3⅓ GRAMS CARDAMOM SEEDS (REMOVED FROM PODS)
7 GRAMS WHOLE FENNEL
1½ GRAMS GROUND CORIANDER
1 GRAM CINNAMON STICK

Pour the gin into a measuring cup. Add the cardamom, fennel, and coriander to the gin and let sit for 4 hours. Add the cinnamon stick and let sit for an additional 1½ hours. Strain into a clean, airtight glass container.

## THYME-INFUSED RUM

8 OUNCES (1 CUP) RUM
2 GRAMS THYME SPRIGS

Pour the rum into a measuring cup. Add the thyme sprigs to the rum. Let sit for 12 hours. Strain into a clean, airtight glass container.

## VANILLA-INFUSED COGNAC

8 OUNCES (1 CUP) COGNAC
1.8 GRAMS VANILLA BEAN POD

Pour the cognac into a measuring cup. Halve the vanilla bean lengthwise and add to the cognac. Let sit for 4 hours. Strain into a clean, airtight glass container.

## VANILLA and SAFFRON–INFUSED BOURBON

8 OUNCES (1 CUP) BOURBON
1.2 GRAMS VANILLA BEAN POD
5 THREADS SAFFRON

Pour the bourbon into a measuring cup. Slice the vanilla bean lengthwise and add to the bourbon with the saffron. Let sit for 4 hours. Strain into a clean, airtight glass container.

## SMOKED

### HICKORY-SMOKED WHITE PEACH PURÉE

30 GRAMS HICKORY WOOD CHIPS, FOR SMOKING
250 GRAMS ORGANIC WHITE PEACHES, PITTED, PEELED, AND CUBED

Place the hickory chips on the bottom of a stainless steel steamer. Put the peach cubes in the upper section of the steamer and cover. Heat on low until the wood chips get very smoky but before they catch flame. Allow the peaches to absorb the smoke. Place the smoked peaches into a blender and blend until smooth. Store the peach purée in a clean, airtight glass container and keep refrigerated.

### HICKORY-SMOKED PINEAPPLE PURÉE

30 GRAMS HICKORY WOOD CHIPS, FOR SMOKING
250 GRAMS WHOLE PINEAPPLE, PEELED, CORED, AND CUBED

Place the hickory chips on the bottom of a stainless steel steamer. Put the pineapple cubes in the upper section of the steamer and cover. Heat on low until the wood chips get very smoky but before they catch flame. Allow the pineapple to absorb the smoke. Place the smoked pineapple in a blender and blend until smooth. Store the pineapple purée in a clean, airtight glass container and keep refrigerated.

### PALO SANTO–SMOKED RUM

5 GRAMS PALO SANTO (1 SMALL STICK)
8 OUNCES (1 CUP) RUM

Place the palo santo into a large stainless steel bowl. Place a slightly smaller stainless steel bowl inside the larger bowl. Fill the smaller bowl with rum. Tent the larger bowl with aluminum foil and heat on a hotplate for 2 minutes until the wood becomes very smoky but before it catches flame. Let the rum sit with the smoke for 1 hour. Store the rum in a clean, airtight glass container.

## DRY MIXES

### CURRY SALT

4½ GRAMS SALT
4½ GRAMS CARDAMOM SEED
4 GRAMS CLOVES
3 GRAMS FENNEL SEED
2 GRAMS TURMERIC
2 GRAMS CUMIN
2 GRAMS CAYENNE

Add all ingredients to a small bowl and grind finely. Store in an airtight container and keep dry.

### GROUND PISTACHIOS MIX

75 GRAMS SHELLED PISTACHIOS
0.2 GRAM GROUND CARDAMOM
0.5 GRAM GROUND ALLSPICE

Grind the pistachios into a fine powder, place in a bowl, and mix with the ground cardamom and allspice. Store in an airtight container and keep dry.

## SAMBUCA AND ANISE SEA SALT

150 GRAMS SEA SALT
2 STAR ANISE PODS
¼ OUNCE SAMBUCA

Add the sea salt and anise to a shallow stainless steel dish. Add the sambuca to a corner of the dish and ignite the sambuca. Carefully stir the flaming sambuca throughout the mixture until the flame burns out. Store in an airtight container and keep dry.

## SESAME AND ANISE SEA SALT

150 GRAMS SEA SALT
8 GRAMS BLACK SESAME SEEDS
2 STAR ANISE PODS
¼ OUNCE ABSINTHE

Add the dry ingredients to a shallow stainless steel dish. Add the absinthe to a corner of the dish and ignite the absinthe. Carefully stir the flaming absinthe throughout the mixture until the flame burns out. Store in an airtight container and keep dry.

SELECTED BIBLIOGRAPHY: Arnold, Dave. *Liquid Intelligence: The Art and Science of the Perfect Cocktail*. New York: W. W. Norton & Company, 2014. • De Vos, Paula. "Apothecaries, Artists, and Artisans: Early Industrial Material Culture in the Biological Old Regime." *Journal of Interdisciplinary History* 45, no. 3 (2015): 277–336. • McGee, Harold. *On Food and Cooking: The Science and Lore of the Kitchen (Completely Revised and Updated)*. New York: Scribner, 2004. • Parsons, Brad Thomas. *Bitters: A Spirited History of a Classic Cure-All, with Cocktails, Recipes, and Formulas*. New York: Ten Speed Press, 2011. • Rogers, Adam. *Proof: The Science of Booze*. New York: Mariner Books/Houghton Mifflin Harcourt, 2014. • Rogers, Kara. *Out of Nature: Why Drugs from Plants Matter to the Future of Humanity*. University of Arizona Press, 2012. • Stewart, Amy. *The Drunken Botanist: The Plants That Create the World's Great Drinks*. Chapel Hill: Algonquin Books of Chapel Hill, 2013.

## ACKNOWLEDGMENTS

Our agent, Coleen O'Shea of the Allen O'Shea Literary Agency, has been a joy to work with and much appreciation for her support and guidance.

The Harper Design team has made this a wonderful collaborative process. We are grateful to Marta Schooler, publisher, and our editor, Tricia Levi. Thanks also to Lynne Yeamans, Soyolmaa Lkhagvadorj, Katherine Lindsey Haigler, and Suzette Lam.

Many thanks to Raphael Geroni for his gorgeous book design and to our talented photographers: Art Gray, Max Milla, and Johnny Miller.

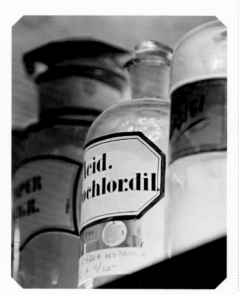

We greatly appreciate the Apotheke team's contributions to the book: Nicolas O'Connor, Seth Bulkin, Andrew Hood, Yibran Rodriguez, and Ryan O'Connor. With gratitude to all of our amazing staff who make the magic happen. And to Ian Martin for his creativity in the assistance of the interior design.

### FROM CHRISTOPHER

I'd like to thank my parents for raising me in Indiana, and raising me right. Thanks to Erica Brod for her thorough and dedicated work with this book. A special thanks to my sister, Heather Tierney, for having the vision to sign an unprecedented lease in New York's Chinatown that is responsible for the brand's genesis.

### FROM ERICA

Thanks to Christopher Tierney for this amazing opportunity. I'm eternally grateful to my husband, Scott Brod, my rock throughout. My mom was an unwavering source of support (and babysitting), as were neighbors the Chmutovs and the O'Gradys. Many thanks to friends who gave suggestions: you know who you are! I'm also grateful to my past and present writing mentors.

# INDEX

## ABOUT THE AUTHORS

CHRISTOPHER TIERNEY, Apotheke / Founder & Designer, was an artist-entrepreneur and an explorer at heart, whose appreciation and connection to the natural world was always an effervescent part of his spirit and inspiration. For all his projects, he experienced an indescribable exhilaration when he would lock onto a concept and allow the laws of attraction to direct the creative process. "I find the universe can be quite generous at times…and it's in these moments I feel most alive," he said.

Christopher discovered the Indiana University woodshop while majoring in biology. During his final semester, he spent most his free time in the carpentry shop designing and fabricating a series of furniture pieces that would earn him a scholarship to the Academy of Art, San Francisco. His studies in Interior Architecture and Design cut the path for his design career, and he formed the design label TIER.

Soon after, Christopher began creating Apotheke on Doyers Street. Since its opening in 2008, it has become his most significant creative endeavor, and he remained the proprietor until his passing in 2022.

Christopher led the design and branding for numerous hospitality and residential clients. Part of TIER Creative's ethos was that it was mandatory to be involved in all stages of the design and process, and to form the brand identity through hands-on artisanal finishes. Christopher believed that function should marry form, and employed a multidisciplined design approach that nurtured inviting works of art. He was excited by the challenge to create atmospheres where people experience a visceral sense of emotion, have meaningful conversation, and grow relationships. With an original style, deep knowledge of craft, and affinity for detail, Christopher delivered seamless results across a diverse conceptual range. In addition, Christopher's experience as proprietor added a unique value for clients from his thorough perspective as both the designer and the developer. His creative work has been featured in numerous publications and has been awarded for aesthetic prestige both domestically and internationally.

**Christopher will be remembered by his friends and family as an arbiter of culture, a student of nature, a creative spirit, and a visionary.**

ERICA BROD is a New Jersey–based writer and editor. As the director of marketing and content for AlphaOmega, she created and managed all of the startup company's content and social media. Among other freelance projects, she has served as a freelance writer's assistant for Wild Obscura and a contributing writer for *The Somerville Times*.

Before moving to NYC, Erica worked for five years at Ceres, an advocate for sustainability leadership based in Boston, Massachusetts, where she cowrote and edited reports and a wide range of other items. She graduated from Brown University with a Master of Public Policy and from the University of Massachusetts at Amherst with a Bachelor of Arts in Sociology.

After living on Doyers Street in an apartment above Apotheke for a few years, she now lives near the Jersey Shore with her husband, Scott, and their daughter, Skye.